Lyme Disease Supercharge

*The Revolutionary Approach
to Getting Better
When All Else Fails*

Bryan Rosner

Edited by Christa Upton
Foreword by Daniel Cagua-Koo, PMA, MD, MPH

Order additional copies from: www.lymebook.com

BioMed Publishing Group

PO Box 9012

South Lake Tahoe, CA 96158

For comments or questions, please email us at bmpublish@gmail.com. You can also call us at the number listed at www.lymebook.com

ISBN 978-1-7337645-0-6

Disclaimer

I am not a doctor. This book is not intended as medical advice. Consult your licensed physician for medical advice. This book is not intended to prevent, diagnose, treat, or cure any medical condition. This book is written to express my personal opinion and experiences only.

I am not a professional mold expert. The references in this book to mold problems in homes or human bodies is based on my own informal, uncertified research and experience, and is not to be construed as professional advise. Please consult a licensed mold professional for advice related to mold problems.

This book is written to share my own informal and unprofessional opinions, observations, and research. It should not be treated as a professional resource. Consult licensed physicians and licensed mold experts for professional information.

ACKNOWLEDGMENTS

Of course, there are really too many people to list here.

God is at the top of the list, and I am thankful that He guided us through this journey.

I want to thank my wife, without whom this book – and my own healing – would never have been possible. While my wife was never as mold-sick as I was, she was affected by mold. I've always been grateful for this, because it allowed us to remain a team. She understood what I was going through. I love you Leila, you are the best wife ever!

I would also like to thank my parents and my entire Tahoe community, who helped launch us onto our mold avoidance RV road trip and journey.

And of course, Lisa and Erik, who pioneered this approach to healing, and without whom none of this would be possible.

I would also like to thank all of the more experienced mold avoiders who helped me learn the path to healing. Jumping into this fight is chaotic and difficult for anyone who attempts it, and I don't think I would have made it if it weren't for the help of people who spent their time guiding me. Especially, Simcha, Nikki, Christi (who supported my wife), and many others.

**Don't miss our new books of interest
to Lyme and Mold patients!**

Visit www.lymebook.com to see our complete selection.
Our books are recommended by patients
and physicians worldwide.

To join our mailing list,
please visit www.lymebook.com/newsletter

TABLE OF CONTENTS

Foreword

By Daniel Cagua-Koo, PMA, MD, MPH

Bryan Rosner has written a phenomenally informative and entertaining book detailing his mold avoidance journey. The message in the book is important for EVERYONE who struggles with chronic illness and who has been given a diagnosis of various idiopathic (unknown cause) diseases, like CFS (Chronic Fatigue Syndrome), ME, MCAD, Chronic Lyme, and others.

Through sharing his mold avoidance journey, Bryan is highlighting the impact of biological mold toxins, both indoors and outdoors. Exposures to mold toxins, both indoors and outdoors, are often the main unrecognized cause of chronic illness. Avoiding both indoor toxins and outdoor biological toxins is part of the mold avoidance journey. Unfortunately, understanding of outdoor biological toxin exposure is not widely recognized by the integrative health care community.

Bryan Rosner's journey is particularly insightful, because of his expertise in Lyme and co-infections. He describes treatments for Lyme and co-infections and heavy metal chelation in the context of mold avoidance. He masterfully describes the dynamic interaction between mold toxicity and chronic infections and demonstrates the far superior outcomes when he combines mold avoidance with the various Lyme and co-infections therapies that he has written about in his prior books.

The most powerful therapeutic treatment for a wide variety of illnesses is removing yourself from toxic mold exposures (both indoors and outdoors) and planting yourself in a good location.   I have personally been made seriously ill by these toxins and have recovered most of my health by doing mold avoidance (again, both indoor and outdoor biological toxins) as well as incorporating supportive therapies. Basically, locations matter. They matter a lot. These are the incredible insights we have learned from Erik Johnson, a pioneer in mold avoidance who you will read about in Bryan's book.

Daniel Cagua-Koo, PMA, MD, MPH
Founder, River of Life Medical
www.riveroflifemedical.org

Part I:

ANOTHER CHANCE
AT LIFE

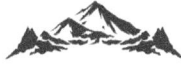

Chapter 1

A RADICAL NEW APPROACH

The approach described in this book has helped many super-sick people to recover some or all of their health, when all else has failed. You may be skeptical of this claim, and wonder why more people aren't using this supposed amazing treatment. After all, if it works so well, why aren't more people talking about it online? How could it possibly be a secret? The answer is that understanding this approach requires a very open mind, and a new paradigm.

This is a book about mold and how it keeps Lyme disease patients sick. However, I did not want to include the word "mold" in the title of the book. Why not? Because most of you wouldn't read it if I did.

Most people feel that mold is old news in the Lyme disease world. It is already well-established that mold is a huge factor in the Lyme disease recovery process. Many people are already aware of this, and feel that they have already dealt with mold. Or, they think that mold isn't that big of an issue for them. Personally I made both of these false assumptions. And it wasn't even my fault. The mold information distributed by modern Lyme disease experts is, in many cases, flat-out wrong, or at least inadequate, and can lead people into a false sense of comfort and make them think that mold isn't really their issue or that they have already dealt with their mold. In this book, I am going to introduce you to a new paradigm that is so radical and so non-conventional that it usually takes people being on their deathbeds before they consider it. That was the case with me: I was literally on my deathbed. I thought I had dealt with mold. It is my hope that you will consider this paradigm before you get as sick as I was. And remember, I am a full-time Lyme disease researcher and journalist. So if I can miss this information, so can you!

This book is based on a little-known, radical view of mold that completely changed my life and rescued me from being a dying person. The approach this book describes is commonly known as "extreme mold avoidance," but as you'll see, it is more nuanced than you might guess. The mold information I found in normal sources didn't help me; it lulled me to sleep so that I believed mold wasn't my issue, because I had "already tried that." Ask yourself how many Lyme disease sufferers you know who are still sick but have "already dealt with mold." I bet it's a lot. The truth is that if you know how to look, you might find that mold is the root cause of a lot more of your health problems than you realize. Extreme mold avoidance isn't just a closer look at mold and how it can keep us sick. It is an entirely *different* paradigm than the normal mold treatment procedures that dominate medicine today.

But most of my readers are Lyme disease patients, so they may be wondering why I am talking to them about mold. They may think that mold is *part* of their problem, but that Lyme disease is a bigger part. Well, I titled this book "Lyme Disease Supercharge" because people who follow the approach described in this book gain the ability to supercharge their Lyme healing process. The approach in and of itself can provide an incredible level of healing, but what's more, it also allows the other therapies you are using to work much, much better. Exponentially better.

When I began following the approach in this book, my "Lyme disease" went from being a huge monster that didn't want to stay in it's cage at all, no matter what I did, to being a tame little wimpy mouse, who would sit down and be quiet if I just took a few drops of a simple herb. Extreme mold avoidance has been the secret weapon that has made this possible.

The approach discussed in this book treats mold toxins as the "master" toxin. The earth is a polluted, toxic place, and we can't avoid all toxins, so we have to pick and choose which ones are most important to avoid. By avoiding the master toxin (mold), many people, including myself, have noticed that our reactivity and the harm that results from exposure to other toxins, foods, or allergens, radically decreases. Our infections dissipate, our brain starts working again, and we get healthy and strong...all by putting the most focus on the master toxin and doing whatever it takes to avoid it. How do we know which mold to avoid, and how much of it we can tolerate? Keep reading to find out.

So, buckle your seatbelt, open your mind, and get ready to discover a whole new paradigm. It is as strange as it is powerful, and it is a secret weapon to regaining health when all else fails.

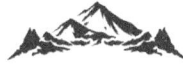

Chapter 2

LYME'S DIRTY SECRET

I almost titled this book "Lyme's Dirty Secret." Because I really do believe this information is a secret. I've been researching this stuff full-time for decades, and even I didn't know about this. Not because the information itself is so hard to find, but because a massive paradigm shift is necessary in order to accept the information. The fact that mold is already so well-known in the Lyme disease world further adds to the obscurity of the approach described in this book, because people feel that they have already read about or addressed their mold issues.

Before talking more about the approach, I want to share a few more examples of how the typical mold information is inadequate:

❖ Many people are told they have Lyme disease and mold toxicity, and they are instructed to take a drug called cholestyramine to detox. Yet, many of these people are unable to tolerate this drug, due to factors that some doctors aren't willing to face. This is what happened to me. Or, they can tolerate the drug, but still don't get better.

❖ People are told to try to find mold-free housing in order to heal. Yet, the tools provided to help people assess their housing, and find new housing, often don't work, and leave people sick. Tragically, if people employ these tools and remain sick, they are told that "mold has been dealt with" and their problem must be something else. This is probably the most important factor that makes the approach in this book different from other mold therapies: the truth that conventionally remediated homes which have been "cleared" as mold free, in many cases, are still not adequately clear of mold for mold sensitive people to heal.

❖ People are not told about the many nuances of mold detox and healing, or about the different framework, or paradigm, that applies to those with mold toxicity. The paradigm is so counter-intuitive, and foreign, that people will never figure it out unless they are given access to special information on the topic. Yet, special information isn't provided by Lyme doctors, beyond a very basic approach to addressing mold toxicity.

❖ People are not told that outdoor air, and the presence of a few types of "special" outdoor molds, may be keeping them sick, no matter how good their indoor environment is. This was the case with me personally!

❖ People are not shown the existence of a massive online community of those who have "failed" normal mold and Lyme treatments, but who are regaining their health through a radical, revolutionary healing approach developed by a person who is one of the prototype cases of Chronic Fatigue Syndrome, Erik Johnson.

❖ People are not told that they have the power to single-handedly change their own destinies. Instead, they are being peddled expensive "treatments," standard "doctor appointments," and "mold tests." The medical establishment is trying to fix this problem with treatments, when it is at its root an environmental problem, that needs to be fixed by changing one's environment. This is not easily done, so I don't fault doctors for doing their best with the tools that they have. But it is my job to tell the truth, and the truth is that mold illness, and often Lyme disease, is an environmental illness that needs to be managed as such.

In short, people don't know that Lyme disease has a dirty little secret. They don't know that mold may still be their problem, even if they've already "treated" their mold. And they don't know just how profound the mold component of this illness is. In fact, it has been observed that almost ALL chronic illnesses involve mold, and each day new studies are being published on various debilitating neurodegenerative diseases which elucidate the mold component.

How do I know all of this? Because I was one of the people who didn't know. And if it can happen to me, it can happen to you. Why? Because I've researched Lyme disease for a living for more than 15 years. If information can slip through my fingers, it can slip through anyone's fingers. My hope is that this book saves you the many years which I lost because I was ignorant of Lyme's dirty secret.

You'll read about my story in this book, and see how Lyme's dirty secret kept me sick for years. And you may even discover that Lyme's dirty little secret is keeping you sick, too.

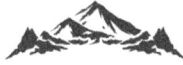

Chapter 3

INFORMATION FOR THE READER

Watch a Video Introduction to My Story

I believe it will be valuable and entertaining for you to watch a 25 minute video I made when we were beginning our mold avoidance adventure. You can find this video on the following website:

www.lymebook.com/extreme-mold-avoidance

In this video, I introduce a number of important concepts in a simple, easy-to-watch fashion. I suggest watching the video before continuing to read this book.

Keeping up-to-date

I will be updating my readers on our mold avoidance journey as new information becomes available and as I become more experienced in mold avoidance. Follow my updates by subscribing to my Anti-Lyme Journal at www.antilyme.com. On this website, I will also be doing mold Q & A's, covering some topics which didn't quite make it into this book, or made it into this book but not in enough detail. You can also sign up to be on my email mailing list, here: www.lymebook.com/newsletter.

The Products and Treatments that Helped Me

I would like to share with you the products, treatments and services which have been most helpful to me, so I am maintaining a website where you can find this information. I have chosen to use a website for this purpose instead of printing them in a book, because the information evolves on a daily basis.

Point your web browser to: www.lymebook.com/favorites

My other Lyme disease books

I've written 5 other books on the topics of Lyme disease, autism, rife machines, and related topics. I've also been involved in publishing more than 20 books by doctors and researchers, on topics including Lyme disease, cancer, mercury poisoning, and alternative medicine. Please visit www.lymebook.com to see these books.

A Note from the Author: Finding a Secret Path to Joy

When you read this book, you may be caught off guard by the extreme measures that some people (including myself) have taken in order to improve their health. You may think these measures are unrealistic, and that there's no way you could possibly pursue them. But moreso, you may think that even if you have the ability to pursue them, you wouldn't even want to.

First, let me point out that not everyone needs to be as extreme as I have been in order to successfully pursue the approach described in this book. Consider my book a case study focusing on a very extreme example of mold avoidance. You may require less extreme avoidance than I required.

For example, some people are able to do mold avoidance and still live in conventional housing, go to work, and keep some semblance of normalcy in their lives.

But to me, that isn't the point. One very surprising discovery I made during pursuit of mold avoidance is that there is a secret source of joy in doing this that I never even knew I wanted. As we live our toxic, modern, imbalanced lives, we are not even aware of the joy and peace that awaits us in pursuing a life that is more in tune with nature and with how our bodies were designed to function. And I'm not talking about some fruit-cake philosophy about singing "Kum ba yah" while dancing in a meadow. I'm talking about something much more fundamental than that. Our very biology and physiology cries out for a deep connection to nature. It is not that we shouldn't partake in the benefits of modern life, it is simply that we should also re-acquaint ourselves with the very environment in which our bodies thrive. Fish are made for water, and humans are made for healthy, balanced, nurturing environments.

In doing mold avoidance, I discovered a deep and peaceful joy which went beyond my wildest dreams. This is something many people will not under-stand until they experience it for themselves. It is also something that takes time to discover, just as it takes time for an alcoholic to detox from their addiction and get past the withdrawal symptoms of leaving alcohol behind.

So, what is this magical thing I'm talking about? It is definitely not just "the beauty of nature," although of course I like that too. The very poignant dis-covery I made doing mold avoidance is that what truly brings us happiness in life, is health. It is not technology, nor "modern civilization," nor living like everyone else lives in our country. If I could feel really, truly healthy by doing something else, and not what I describe in this book, then I would go do that. It is not that I have some kind of obsession with nature. Not at all. I do, however, have an obsession with health.

Yet, some of us have been sick for so long that we don't have a frame of ref-erence for health, and so we use the attractions of modern life as consolation prizes. "I don't feel very good, but at least I can watch a movie," some of us say. But once you experience true health and healing, I think you'll agree with me that the experience of just being healthy brings another level of joy and happiness to your life. And so, once you are reminded of what health feels like (because maybe you've forgotten), then you will no longer see mold avoidance as a sacrifice, but instead, as a gift. And, of course, the fact that the beauty of nature is involved in this (instead of the dreariness of doctors' waiting rooms) is just icing on the cake.

When I first began doing mold avoidance, an experienced mold avoider told me that the cities she considers "likable cities" are the ones in which she feels good. She listed some cities which I would never think of as appealing cities, and told me that since she feels good in these cities, these are her favorite cities. It made no sense to me at the time. But as I began to do mold avoidance and experience healing, I quickly understood what she meant. All of the beautiful, toxic places that I no longer visit, are no longer appealing places to me. After being reminded of what health feels like, I have absolutely no desire to go back to those places and function as a half-alive, half-dead creature that slinks around with a fogged brain, body pain, no motivation, no zest for life.

Currently, the things I find myself really seeking are not outward characteristics in a city or environment, but instead, inward characteristics in my own body. Do I wake up refreshed, happy, peaceful, and ready to tackle the day? Is my mind clear and focused, and my mood light and playful? Does the outdoor air smell fresh and clean to me, and do I have a skip in my step as I get in my car? These are the things which matter to me now, and once you too have experienced them, you'll understand why mold avoidance is a gift, even though it may seem like a burden in the beginning. Our vessels – the bodies in which we travel through this – are really all we have. If these vessels are not functioning well, nothing else matters. This may seem painfully obvious, but the fact is that many of us who have been sick for a long time, forget this. We learn to take pleasure in other things, to settle for less. And there's nothing wrong with that, of course. But once you have a taste of feeling good again, you'll never want to go back.

And so I would like to invite you to think of mold avoidance as a gift. It may not be the kind of gift you thought you wanted to receive, but I think you'll change your mind about that.

I am reminded of my son on his first birthday. My wife's policy is that our children don't get to taste sweets until they turn one. When they turn one, they get to have a birthday cupcake. I remember my son screaming and crying about the cupcake. He didn't know what it was; he had no frame of reference for it. He really thought he wanted something else. He refused to even taste it! I literally had to force feed him. It was hilarious. But finally, when he relented and took a bite, his eyes lit up with delight. Now he knew what a cupcake tasted like! He loved it! How could he have ever made an educated decision about cupcakes, without tasting one? And this is how I feel about the fruits of mold avoidance.

On my YouTube channel, I made a video talking about this subject. You may find it worthwhile to watch. It is called "Making Movements Toward Health." You can find it by doing a Google search for "Lyme Disease Publisher on YouTube," or by visiting www.youtube.com/lymediseasepublisher.

In any case, I wanted to open my book with this message to you. Remember, not everyone needs to be as extreme as I have been in pursuing mold avoidance in order to see results. And, try to remember that any resistance you may feel now about living in harmony with nature is probably not your true soul speaking, but instead, just the part of you which has been forced to adapt to living in a toxic and unhealthy world. Try to give your inner, true voice a chance to speak, even if it is is a faint voice at first. I think you'll be glad you kept an open mind about this. And if you succeed in finally feeling healthy, with a vigorous zest for life, I think you'll agree with me that all else pales in comparison.

Thanks for reading my book, and I hope you find peace, joy, and true health.

Written by Bryan Rosner
In the high mountains of New Mexico in February, 2019.

Chapter 4

THE EXPERTS OF MOLD AVOIDANCE: LISA PETRISON, PhD, AND ERIK JOHNSON

My purpose in writing this book is to introduce you to mold avoidance, and to share with you how it has changed my life. However, my book shouldn't be seen as the "how-to" guide for mold avoidance. For that information, you need to explore the extremely thorough and necessary resources created by Lisa Petrison and Erik Johnson. My book should be seen as a road sign, which points you to their work.

Most of my success in mold avoidance and healing came because of the life-saving information contained in two books which they co-wrote: *The Beginner's Guide to Mold Avoidance* and *Erik on Avoidance*. These books are, in my opinion, mandatory reading. You can find links to these books by visiting: www.lymebook.com/avoidance.

Erik is the "Founding Father" of mold avoidance. He also lives in my hometown of Lake Tahoe and became ill with extreme Chronic Fatigue Syndrome / Myalgic Encephalomyelitis (CFS/ME) in the 1980's. He was the first to propose mold as a causative factor for this illness, and while mainstream medicine ignored him, he regained his health doing what we refer to as "extreme mold avoidance." His guidance and wisdom were mandatory in my own healing journey. I have much gratitude for his work. To read his own personal story, please read his biographical book, *Back from the Edge,* which is also linked from: www.lymebook.com/avoidance. Erik never asked to become famous, but he his now. Thousands of extremely sick people have learned Erik's approach and have regained their health by following it, even after all else has failed. Though Erik was bedridden with CFS in the 1980's, and doctors had no answers for him, he is now back to great health.

As a tradition he began after recovering, he still hikes Mt. Whitney every year, one of the most challenging hikes in the United States. He hikes this mountain as a symbol of his ongoing success with mold avoidance. Yet, doctors and researchers still haven't taken notice, and still refuse to look into Erik's approach for the sickest of patients, who continue to languish in bed from their illnesses, despite all kinds of fancy interventions and medications. Erik's approach remains all-natural and doctor-free, and Erik's success has come completely independent of help from the medical establishment. I've been following Erik's work and I continue to see thank-you notes and success stories pouring in, especially from those people who were so sick that they had already given up and were preparing to die. After a person sees this success over and over, it is easy to develop deep gratitude and respect for Erik.

Lisa Petrison, who has co-written and published Erik's books, deserves great thanks for her efforts. Her organizational skills and motivation to help others led her to expend a huge amount of energy to write and edit these books, and to organize the available information into a very useful and approachable format. As a result of the new "mold avoidance movement," there are now several very active online support communities, as well. You can see which mold support groups are currently active, and find links to join them, by visiting: www.lymebook.com/avoidance.

Lisa studied Erik's discoveries and then added her very unique and insightful experiences into the available knowledge base, and I am very appreciative of Lisa's contribution to the mold avoidance community. She herself has pursued "extreme mold avoidance" for more than 10 years and has amassed an almost unbelievable amount of knowledge on the subject. Lisa herself has also mostly recovered from ME/CFS, as a result of following Erik's approach. Lisa is also the founder of Paradigm Change, an organization focused on the role of mold toxins in chronic illness. The Paradigm Change website is rich with fantastic information that is continuously being updated, so I suggest visiting the website as soon as you can.

If Erik hadn't discovered mold avoidance, and if Lisa hadn't organized and written about it, then tens of thousands of people, including myself, would still be desperately sick.

I believe it would be irresponsible and even dangerous to pursue mold avoidance without first reading the books mentioned above. Also, if you are reading my book and encounter phrases or words that are unfamiliar, you can find their definitions in Lisa and Erik's books. Of course, I will do my best to define most of these terms for you in my book, but reading the other books really is a necessity.

In essence, my book should be seen as my own personal experience with mold avoidance, but Lisa and Erik's books should be seen as the foundational, how-to guides.

What Lisa and Erik discovered is that the way to heal from mold toxicity is not merely to rely on laboratory testing and remediation of one's home or living space. Instead, they discovered that the body itself is our best tool for identifying environments where we can heal, but first, we need to learn to listen to our body and understand the clues it gives us. In some cases, homes which are supposedly clear of mold may actually be keeping us sick. In other cases, the outdoor air may be keeping us sick. I highly recommend reading Lisa's free article online, entitled, *Outdoor Toxins of Particular Relevance to Mold Illness Patients*. This article can be found on her website, www.paradigmchange.me. Probably the easiest way to find it, though, is simply to Google the title of the article which I have just listed here. This article was one of the first of Lisa's writings which I encountered, and it was a life-changing read for me. Let me repeat: EVERYONE should stop what they are doing and go read this article.

By following their approach, we can finally give the body the space it needs to heal. In most cases, what our body actually needs in order to heal is quite different from what mold remediators and laboratory tests tell us. And the best part about this discovery is it empowers people to take control of their own health, by relying exclusively on their own unique and powerfully equipped body to craft a path toward healing. What is remarkable about this approach is that Lisa and Erik have been working to perfect it and turn it into an exact science, and they've mostly succeeded. In fact, they have been studying these concepts for decades, and the rest of us can now benefit from their hard work.

I want to point out that some parts of this book focus on my own personal experiences with mold avoidance, and my interpretation of what was happening to my body. I do not claim that my interpretations and experiences will apply equally to everyone.

Don't forget to go read Lisa and Erik's books!
Find links to them at: www.lymebook.com/avoidance.

Chapter 5

LYME DISEASE SUPERCHARGE

Why did I write another book on Lyme disease? Well, to tell the truth, before this book, I kind of hoped that I could retire from writing Lyme disease books. I had already written five books on Lyme disease, and felt that I didn't have much else to say.

However, apparently God had other plans, because this one may be the most important of the books I've written! And furthermore, the last year of my life has been an unbelievable, extreme, and otherworldly adventure, and I think it makes a great story!

Some people will ask me, "Bryan, if the information in your past books was valid, then why did you need to do mold avoidance? Didn't the treatments you describe in your past books make you well?" It's a good question, and I might as well answer it before going any further.

The answer is that those treatments got me as far as I could go, and even into remission and living a pretty normal life for over a decade. To me, that was a success. But my health always seemed incomplete, like there was some piece I was missing, and there were still unanswered questions about deeper healing. It turns out that the problem wasn't that I was using the wrong treatments or that they didn't work well enough. The problem was that my body eventually became too burdened with mold to completely heal.

I had to learn that no treatment or book, no matter how excellent, can compensate for the damage that mold toxicity can cause. When I was in remission and doing well, I believe that I was very successful in healing from Lyme disease and related conditions, as a direct result of the strategies I have shared in my past books. I do not believe I was exposed to a living environment with mold until later on, when we moved into our most recent home. It was at this time that my health took a slow turn for the worse, and even my old Lyme infections began to re-activate. Though looking back now, I do see that I have been exposed to mold for my whole life, and that mold probably contributed to my susceptibility to Lyme disease in the first place. In particular, I discovered that of all the Lyme disease co-infections, Bartonella is the one that flares up the most when mold toxicity is present.

During my worst mold exposure, in our last house, I wasn't aware that I was being exposed to mold. And this is one reason why so many people think that "mold isn't their issue." During intense and prolonged mold exposure, the body employs a strange and counterintuitive behavior called "masking." People who are "masked" may be living in terrible mold, but the body turns off all perceptible reactions to that mold. A person's senses become blinded to the mold, and they don't realize how bad the mold is. Becoming "unmasked" is one of the main goals of successful mold avoidance, and we'll discuss that shortly.

In Fall of 2017, a professional inspection revealed mold in our crawl space. We had the mold professionally remediated and the inspector issued a clearance certificate, but by that time, the damage to my body had already been done. Interestingly, we had never seen visible mold in our home, and we had no knowledge or awareness of water intrusion or rot. Mold can hide in homes which may lead to a false sense of comfort. Mold can even be inside homes with no history of water intrusion or leaks, due to condensation and other construction issues. So, don't discount the possibility of mold being in your home too quickly!

I think that my underlying Lyme disease contributed significantly to my susceptibility to the mold, even though my Lyme disease was mostly in remission when we moved into that house. And mold had probably also contributed to the reason I had Lyme in the first place, so it was a vicious cycle. Mold and Lyme disease are just very bad actors when they get together, no matter which one you think comes first.

It is also known by mold avoiders that the entire Lake Tahoe area has a particularly bad outdoor mold toxin, which probably contributed to my decline. This toxin is known loosely as Mystery Toxin, and is described in the book, *The Beginner's Guide to Mold Avoidance*. It is also described in the article I mentioned above, *Outdoor Toxins of Particular Relevance to Mold Illness Patients*. Many other locations in the United States are also known to have this toxin, and because it is an outdoor toxin, people may move from home to home, trying to seek a mold-free environment, and not even realize that the outdoor air itself is what is keeping them sick. In fact, the omission of outdoor mold toxins from the standard mold information that most Lyme disease patients have access to is one of the huge problems keeping people sick.

After learning these facts, my family felt that the best course of action was to take a break from the entire Lake Tahoe area, and so even though our house had been remediated, we bought a truck and a travel trailer and hit the road as a family. We left on November 22, 2017. It was hard leaving Lake Tahoe, since it has been my hometown for more than thirty years. At the time I write this, we are still living in our RV, more than a year later. We'll get to that part of the story!

I want to point out that not everyone will need to avoid entire regions in order to heal. It seems to be that only the sickest people need to do this. The best course of action, of course, would be to pursue more moderate mold avoidance before a person becomes super-sick, so that they never reach the point where they need to pursue such extreme avoidance. In other words, an ounce of prevention is worth a pound of cure. One of the basic premises of this book is that *avoiding* mold is even more important than using *treatments* for mold. We'll be talking a lot more about this.

After we hit the road, I rapidly began to improve and again found all the treatments listed in my past books to be the best treatments for me. In that sense, I believe my past books were truly valuable, except that they didn't include the powerful destruction that mold can cause to a person's health; especially a person with Lyme disease. And some of the newer treatments which I've discovered since those books were published are included in this new book, so you can learn about them and consider whether they may be helpful to you.

The ability of the old treatments to start working again is why I titled this book "Lyme Disease Supercharge." In simple terms, this book doesn't negate or overrule all the other treatments I've written about. Instead, mold avoidance simply allows those treatments to work better. Much better. Exponentially better. So if you simply aren't getting better no matter what you do, this may be part of your answer. Your Lyme disease treatments may be just fine, but your level of mold exposure and toxicity may be preventing them from helping you. One mold expert I follow has said that mold avoidance is a leverage point for other treatments to work better. I like this explanation.

To further illustrate this concept, consider what happened to me. During my decline in that house prior to the remediation, none of the "good old" Lyme treatments worked anymore. I kept doing the same thing over and over, doing what used to work, and it was useless. I should have woken up and realized there was something else going on, but I didn't, for a long time, and I got sicker and sicker. After all, it isn't in the American culture to assume or even consider the idea that our housing and belongings could be keeping us sick. It was such a paradigm shift that it completely escaped me. Animals move from place to place in the wilderness to seek ideal living conditions, but humans stubbornly insist upon living in the same abode for decades or sometimes even longer.

But, you say, "mold is already widely recognized in the Lyme disease community as a causative factor in Lyme disease, so why do we need this book?" Well, the truth is, that I have long known about mold and even pursued various mold treatments, and none of it helped at all. Currently available information on mold isn't *wrong*, it is just *inadequate*. This book is an attempt to bridge the gap.

My house was a newer, well-maintained home with no visible signs of mold and no history of leaks or water damage. We had no reason to suspect mold in our home, or our entire town, for that matter. Even though I was able to successfully remediate my home and sell it, the damage had already been done to my body, and the way out of the maze was much more complex than simply moving into a different home.

Once a person's body has become damaged by mold, even a remediated house may not be adequate for healing. The home may be OK for "normal people," but not for people who have fallen into the depths of mold illness. Mycotoxins can be absorbed into all the building and finish materials throughout a house, as well as a person's belongings. A more extreme approach was clearly needed, an approach which you won't read about much online or hear about at your Lyme Doctor's office. It is this more extreme approach that I tell you about in this book. And I believe it is extremely important information. If the typical mold information were good enough, I wouldn't have written this book at all.

But I was also one of the many people who didn't even realize that the outdoor air was just as big of a problem for me as my indoor living space. Clearly, I was experiencing a heightened sensitivity to mold which "normal people" don't experience. Thousands of normal people live in the Tahoe area and are perfectly healthy. Lyme and mold doctors rarely, if ever, acknowledge the importance of outdoor mold toxins, nor do they recognize or even know about some of the finer points of mold avoidance which to me have been nothing short of lifesaving. To people who are very sick, these details mean everything, and may mean the difference between healing and remaining debilitated. It is this "next level" of mold information that I think people need to discover.

It turns out that I'm not the only one who has experienced the inadequacies of modern mold information. The Mold Avoiders Facebook Group run by Lisa Petrison has over 11,000 members now, and many of them have recovered a great deal of their health after not having benefited much from most of the "normal" mold therapies. And so I believe this information is important and is worthy of a new book. So, this book will share with you the mold information which actually helped me. And I think you'll agree with me that this information *isn't yet* in other readily available Lyme disease books and resources. So, that is why I wrote this book.

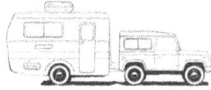

Chapter 6

DREAMING OF RV LIFE – A MESSAGE FROM MY SUBCONSCIOUS

I began daydreaming about the RV lifestyle long before I knew anything about mold.

It was summer, 2016. I didn't know it, but this was about the time when we think the mold issue began in our home. The following winter would prove to be the biggest winter in Tahoe's history, and inflict even further damage and carnage on the Tahoe homes and infrastructure, which would be covered in more than ten feet of snow.

I began surfing the web late at night, looking at RVs and travel trailers. My wife was resistant to the idea of getting one. She thought I was crazy. She preferred tent camping, and I actually did too. But still, there was something about RVs I couldn't shake. I dreamed of family vacations to the coast, and to warmer climates during the winter months, to lush forests. There was just something about RV life that called to me.

Looking back now, it is clear to me that we liked tent camping so much because it got us out of mold exposure. We frequently told our friends how good we felt while tent camping, and we were often met with blank stares.

I didn't tell my wife at the time, but my seemingly innocent, midlife crisis dreams, went beyond just owning an RV. I daydreamed of selling everything we owned, moving into an RV, and traveling indefinitely. We had friends at the time who were also enthralled with this dream, and we used to spend long evenings chatting and scheming. But for me, it was like an obsession.

Looking back, I now know that my body subconsciously, intuitively longed to get away. FAR away. Away from not just my house, but from my city, and from civilization. Or, "civilidevastation," as Erik Johnson calls it. It turns out that mold toxins are often saturating the air of not just moldy homes, but also many cities and civilized areas.

I mean, why wasn't I just daydreaming about exotic hotels in Hawaii or Alaska? No, I was very specifically obsessed with the idea of being in an RV, far away from manmade structures. My body knew what I needed before this need bubbled up to a conscious level. I mean I was literally dreaming and fantasizing about a life which seemed so unusual and impossible, but a life which would very soon become our reality. I almost titled this book "Mold Avoidance Road Trip," but later realized that this wasn't really a road trip; it was a new way of life.

What's so special about an RV, versus a hotel? Well, at the time, I wouldn't have been able to tell you. Or at least, I wouldn't have been able to give a succinct, thorough answer, because it was just an intuitive longing. But now, after having lived in an RV full time for over a year, I can come up with some pretty important distinctions. Distinctions which, apparently, my subconscious was aware of long ago:

❖ The RV lifestyle is versatile. It allows for travel and movement, and experimentation with different climates, outdoor environments, and biomes.

❖ The RV lifestyle is an outdoor lifestyle. Not only is the living space inside too small to want to dwell in for very long, RV's are also parked in outdoor spaces. Think about it: When you live in a home, hotel, or apartment, the outdoors is usually not right outside your door. You will find parking lots, driveways, decks, hallways, garages, and other man-made structures outside your door. With an RV, in contrast, you can park in nature-centric areas and literally step outside into the great outdoors. It turns out that one of the silver linings of this "extreme mold avoidance" stuff is that it is best pursued in pristine, remote outdoor areas.

❖ The RV lifestyle is minimal. It is much easier to monitor and take care of a very small vessel, and in our RV, I can do most of this work by myself, taking extra care that there are no water intrusions or other mold-promoting conditions. Belongings are kept to a minimum because of necessity. Whereas, controlling the environment inside rented hotel rooms is unrealistic (you'll learn why as you continue reading).

❖ The RV lifestyle is also supportive of intimate, close family time and relationships, which I think our society is short on in this age of everyone always on the run to school and extracurricular activities. (We ended up homeschooling our kids during the trip).

❖ While an RV does allow you to penetrate deep into nature and get away from civilization, it isn't "roughing it." It has all the creature comforts and attributes of modern shelter that keep adults and children safe and secure from the elements, and all the amenities that allow for a modern lifestyle. In this way, it is the perfect compromise between the two extremes of tent camping and living in a conventional home. As I mentioned, spending time in a "good" or "pristine" location is a huge part of the recovery process from mold illness.

❖ Living in an RV is a great place to embark upon what I refer to as "mold avoidance kindergarten," where big mistakes are relatively low-consequence, because RV's can be traded in a lot more easily than homes.

❖ Living and traveling in an RV allows you to compare different outdoor environments, without the variable of changing indoor environments. I can't emphasize this point enough. When you move from city to city and feel different in each place (a concept known as the "locations effect"), if you are staying in hotel rooms, it is difficult to know what changed: The hotel or the outdoor air? In contrast, changes noticed while living in an RV are always changes in the outdoor environment, because you know that your indoor living space is the same from place to place. This turned out to be an invaluable learning tool for us, as some areas had outdoor toxins which kept us just as ill as indoor mold. In fact, without this benefit of RV life, I am positive that we wouldn't have healed.

Somehow, my soul and spirit and physical body knew we needed these things before my conscious mind realized it.

I don't think we would have ever pursued this lifestyle, had we not been forced to do it. I would have never had the guts to break ties with the "ordinary" life. And, possibly, the mold that we were living in was actually controlling my mind, keeping me in a mold prison as a vessel for the mold to grow and proliferate. It is scientifically known that many microorganisms exert mind control on their hosts in order to gain a survival advantage, and I believe mold is no different...more on this later.

My obsession with buying an RV was uncontainable. It just grew and grew, and I never knew why. I believe these intuitive longings and messages from our subconscious minds should not be ignored. In fact, as I mentioned earlier, people who are mold sick are often "masked" to the mold, meaning they are not aware that they are living in mold. So, subtle, subconscious messages may indeed be all that you have alerting you to the fact that there is a problem; a BIG problem in your life and health and housing.

Later, after I became "unmasked" and could sense the mold in our home, I began to have dreams and visions of the desert. Literally. I would wake up in the middle of the night and do Google searches for images of the desert, and I would literally just stare at those images for hours in the middle of the night. I would later learn that Erik Johnson spent a lot of time healing in the desert; or the Godforsaken Desert (GFD), as he called it. But it would also turn out that many equally pristine locations could be found in areas with humidity. The commonality appeared to be getting away from civilization. It turns out that many civilized areas, including homes and buildings and infrastructure, are built with toxic chemicals that feed mold and cause it to produce the worst possible sorts of toxins. So the GFD is actually any place that is mostly untouched by human developments, and where the natural microbiome is fairly close to how God intended it to be.

If all of the information in this book so far seems far-fetched or sci-fi, I don't blame you. Even if you are open minded, you may be incredibly skeptical by now. This skepticism is what keeps people from entertaining this new paradigm, often until it is too late. What do I mean by too late? You'll read about that in the next chapter. Too late often means people are "crawling out of their homes and sleeping in the cars" according to Erik Johnson. That very thing happened to me, don't let yourself get to that point!

You aren't in Kansas anymore, Dorothy. The path to healing from this strange condition became an entire new paradigm that took me months to begin to understand.

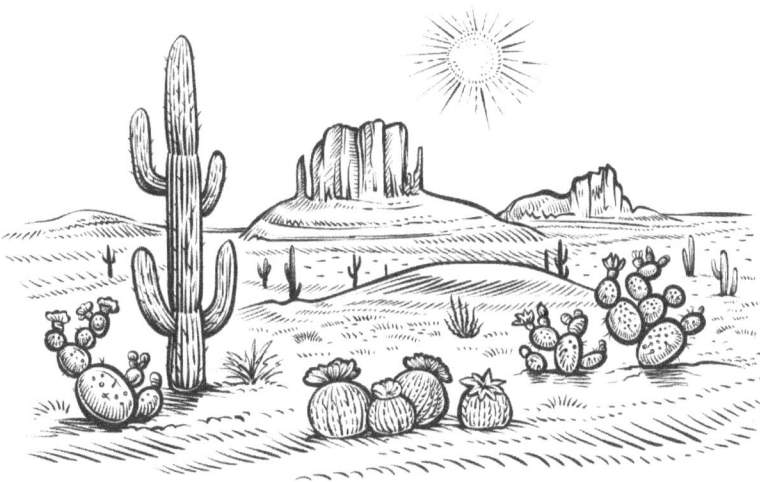

Chapter 7

MY RUDE AWAKENING

In the mold avoider world, we use the term "unmasked" to describe what happens when a person who previously didn't notice any mold in their environment, all of a sudden has a violent and intolerable reaction to mold that has been right under their nose for years. Unmasking usually occurs after you've taken a break from being in your home, and a break from being surrounded by your contaminated belongings.

When constantly exposed to mold, the immune system basically gives up and no longer tells you there's any danger. This is referred to as being "masked." While being masked may seem more pleasant than being unmasked (because being unmasked means experiencing more nasty reactions to mold), being masked causes you to not avoid the molds that are hurting you, hence perpetuating immune suppression and multi-organ dysfunction within the body. Think of being masked as having a tasteless poison put in your food every morning; it has no taste so you don't know it is harming you. And being unmasked is like all of a sudden being able to taste that poison. Wouldn't you prefer to be able to taste the poison, so you can spit it out?

So it is sort of a mixed bag, with pros and cons, when it comes to becoming unmasked. But most people in this situation are so ill, that becoming unmasked and facing the challenge of mold avoidance is still a MUCH more desirable option than not experiencing mold reactions but continuing to live in exposure to mold and getting progressively sicker and closer to death. In fact, if I had to summarize the approach discussed in this book succinctly, it would be the following: The goal is to become unmasked and then heal by avoiding the toxins that we react to. It's that simple. As healing continues, reactivity at first seems to increase, as a person enters the "intensification" phase, and then eventually reactivity decreases.

This is the main thing that separates this book from other information on healing from mold. Normal mold approaches involve using laboratory tests to determine if an environment is free of mold. But the approach described in this book, instead, encourages people to first spend time in a very clear location in order to become unmasked, and then to use the body's own reactions as the "test" to determine whether particular environments are safe enough in which to heal. The approach in this book also asserts that when not clear of these toxins, the body's detox processes are shut down. When detox is shut down, toxins will continue to build up inside the body, no matter how many herbs, supplements, or therapies are employed. Read *The Beginner's Guide to Mold Avoidance* for more on these concepts.

When people suspect they may be masked and wish to become unmasked, a "mold avoidance sabbatical" can be utilized. This is essentially a several week vacation from your home and stuff. Some people choose to buy cheap new clothing, rent a car, and tent camp or stay at a hotel in an area which is known to have good air, as a way of pursuing the sabbatical.

The immune system and detox processes then have a chance to normalize and catch up, and when you return to your stuff and home, if it is moldy, the immune system then goes crazy and reacts strongly. Killing infections and co-infections also helps some people in the process of becoming unmasked. In particular, a treatment known as ten pass ozone can be helpful in this process. I discuss ten pass ozone more in this chapter, and in other chapters throughout the book. Ten pass ozone has been a foundational treatment for me over the past year, and I've had over 25 treatments done.

Please note that undertaking a mold sabbatical requires careful thought and preparation. Instructions for doing this properly can be found in the book, *The Beginner's Guide to Mold Avoidance.*

For people struggling with the concept of a mold sabbatical, there is a very good analogy that will help you understand it. Think about gluten intolerance. Many people who regularly eat gluten may not even know it is harming them. They are "masked" to the damage that gluten is doing to their bodies. It is only *after* gluten is removed from the diet for an extended period, do they then notice the damage gluten does when they return to gluten-containing foods later on and notice dramatic reactions. It is a very similar thing we are trying to achieve with a mold avoidance sabbatical; that is, to be away from mold long enough to begin to actually notice the damage mold is causing us in the form of perceptible reactions. Of course, avoiding gluten is much easier than avoiding your home, all of your belongings, and, in some cases, your entire city or region. But the concept, nonetheless, is the same.

In September of 2017, after living for 9 years in our most recent home, I was the sickest I had ever been. I had a co-infection presence – likely a Bartonella abscess – in my jugular vein in the side of my neck which exploded and caused deranged blood flow inside my brain, leading to many M.S. like symptoms and horrible psychiatric symptoms. I experienced one continuous panic attack which came out of nowhere and lasted over 5 months. I also had many other creeping health problems and worsening of my Lyme infections. I was mostly homebound, and months went by in a blur which felt like days. The previous year, in Fall of 2016, I acquired a tetanus infection in my foot that wouldn't go away and became debilitating for months and months and never completely resolved. I visited the ER five times in two months. Being in this condition was a big change for me, since I had been in remission and feeling great for most of the prior decade.

As I write this 9 months later, I am feeling much better, the best I've felt in years. Two days ago, I went on a 15 mile bike ride with 2,000 vertical feet of elevation gain.

I would later learn that mold spores are most active in the Fall, and this accounted for my typical Fall flareups. Erik Johnson calls it the "November Effect". I used to think that the Lyme bacteria were more active in the Fall, but the fact that many mold avoiders experience these fall flareups – even mold avoiders who don't have Lyme disease – taught me that there was some independent variable here; a variable which isn't specific only to Lyme disease.

A year later, in Fall, 2017, when I was very sick and running out of options, I went to see Dr. Mary Ellen Shannon, MD, of the Irvine, CA, Center for New Medicine, for a promising therapy known as ozone ten pass. On my YouTube channel, *LymeDiseasePublisher*, you can watch a video in which I am interviewing Dr. Shannon live while undergoing an ozone ten pass treatment.

At this point, I had no idea that mold was affecting me. I was still "masked." I had used ozone in many of its home therapy forms, including ozonated water, ozone insufflations, and ozone injections. Of all the treatments available to me, ozone seemed like the most helpful at the time, and so I hypothesized that the much more powerful ten pass method would prob-ably be good for me. In addition to the aforementioned YouTube video, there is also an article about my experience with ten pass ozone on my blog, www.antilyme.com.

The truth is, I was literally on death's door when I went down to see Dr. Shannon. It was kind of a last-ditch effort. I was even thinking about how to say goodbye to my family and children. My wife and I had many conver-sations about this.

I underwent about 5 or 6 ozone treatments with Dr. Shannon. After the second or third one, I became violently unmasked to mold. I believe this occured due to a combination of the ozone ten pass treatments, as well as being away from my moldy home, car and belongings. The crazy thing about this story is that at the time, I had no idea what unmasking was, and I hadn't even considered that mold was affecting me. I guess it is safe to say that I wasn't experiencing the placebo effect in this mold stuff, since I didn't even know it existed! I thought that I had already dealt with my mold issues.

I also didn't know what a mold sabbatical was, and didn't know that I had accidentally embarked on one by flying down to see Dr. Shannon and leaving most of my belongings behind. Essentially, I stumbled into becoming unmasked.

As divine providence would have it, that trip was the turning point for me.

In the middle of my time in Irvine, for no apparent reason, the hotel room I happened to be staying in suddenly reeked of mold and I could no longer be inside the room for more than 10 minutes. This, despite the fact that the room hadn't even bothered me at all for the first week! I hurriedly packed up my room and moved to a hotel across town that felt better to me, despite that hotel being almost three times as expensive. I instantly became incredibly driven to avoid mold. I told my wife on the phone, "there's something weird that just happened to me with mold, I don't really know what is going on." But that was the last thought I gave it, as at the time, I wasn't really focusing on mold as a part of my recovery.

Later, in reflecting on what happened, I realized that this might have been the strangest thing I had ever experienced. A hotel room that had been fine for me all of a sudden became torture to be inside. I could barely even stay long enough to pack up my belongings. I think I left a few articles of clothing behind because I couldn't bear to take one more breath in that room. I remember literally holding my breath while packing up the room.

After finishing up my ozone treatments, I flew to Monterey, CA, where I met up with my parents, wife, and kids for a long-planned family vacation.

This entire time, I was extremely ill and suffering from moderate dementia.

When my wife picked me up from the Monterey airport after my ozone treatments were finished, she came in our family minivan, and the minivan reeked of a horrible odor I had never smelled before. I was absolutely certain that something really bad had happened to the minivan while I was gone, and I quizzed my wife over and over about it. Again, I was becoming unmasked to the mold toxicity in the van, but I didn't realize it. The mold had been in the van last time I saw the van, but I was "masked" at that time.

I started tearing the van apart, literally removing inside carpet and other components, like a crazy person. I was just tearing the thing apart. My wife was horrified. I finally identified what I felt to be the source: my 3 year old's carseat. As we all know, kids drop food and drink on their carseats, and I now believe that this was the primary source of mold in the car, though the rest of the car turned out to be pretty toxic as well (we ended up selling the vehicle a few months later). When I demanded we immediately buy a new carseat, my wife was extremely confused (and so was I!). I was acting like a crazy person. Crazy, at least, until one understands unmasking. We ended up at a Target at 11pm while I ran in and got a new carseat. It was an emergency. That is how badly the odor was affecting me.

When we got home from our trip, back to Lake Tahoe, I began feeling weird as we entered the Tahoe basin. Again, I wasn't focused on mold or toxins at the time, so I only really realize this in retrospect. Then, I took one step into my home and felt even more strange. This is a home I had lived in for 9 years without noticing any strange feelings or odors. Later that evening, I became completely intolerant of my home. When I went to bed, I began to shake and convulse and with each breath, I was inhaling what felt like a toxic gas. I was SURE that someone poisoned my home while I was gone! It was such an extreme change that it was impossible for me to believe that my body changed while I was gone, not the home. In retrospect, I am sort of glad that I hadn't heard of the concept of unmasking yet, because it validates this experience more to me. I was certainly not making this up. And the steps we were about to take certainly required a high degree of confidence, conviction and belief.

I tried to sleep in the guest bedroom. It wasn't better. I slept from 2am to morning time out in the car. Yes, in the car. It was in the 20's that night. That's how ill my house made me. And you won't believe this...after that evening, I've not spent more than a total of about 10 hours back in that home, and I haven't ever slept there again. Can you imagine that...coming home from a vacation and basically never setting foot in your home again. The ten hours accounts for time I had to spend back at the home cleaning it out and moving my home office materials out. I slept at my parents house during that transition, and each time I went back to my home, I got incredibly ill. I could feel toxins all over the home; I could perceive them just as strongly as if someone had sprayed the air and my belongings with perfume or cologne. Only these toxins felt like things I had never before encountered. I could sense mold toxins covering every millimeter of my entire home. I'm not kidding.

We hired a professional industrial hygienist to test our home. He did in fact discover a widespread mold problem in the crawl space. In a funny way, this was a relief to us. We weren't crazy after all. We paid to have the home professionally remediated, after which it was re-tested and found to be clear. It is important to point out here that if someone is already made sick by mold, then conventional testing and remediation methods may not be enough to make an environment safe for them. So even if your home tests low for mold or you have it remediated and the professionals say it is clear, if you are in the portion of the population that is sensitive to mold toxins, then you still can't rule out mold as a possible cause of your illness. The house may be safe for the "normal" population, but not for you. We decided that because of my Lyme disease and sensitivity to mold, that we wanted to move on from the home. So we completed the recommended remediation, re-tested the home to confirm that the remediation was successful, and sold it, disclosing the prior mold problem to the buyers.

I was so motivated to leave my home that we were moved out within 2 weeks. Completely moved out. Imagine that. With no prior planning or intention, we moved out of our home of 9 years in two weeks. We sold most of our belongings at a steep loss. It was sheer desperation. Almost all of our belongings were so contaminated with mycotoxins that we couldn't even keep essential items like my wife's purse, my work computer, clothing, my wife's wedding dress, and other items. Our friends and family who helped us move did not feel any reactions from our belongings, which assured me that it was our damaged bodies that couldn't handle these exposures, not necessarily the general public.

As an aside, it is recommended that people put most of this stuff in storage rather than getting rid of it, because it may become tolerable at a later date and brash, rushed decisions aren't always the best decisions. Sometimes, people heal enough that they can come back to their belongings later and save some of them.

We debated the ethics of selling our items to other families, but then realized that many of our healthy friends lived in similar homes in Tahoe without a problem. Not everyone has mold illness. We did disclaim to possible buyers that these items had come from a home with a mold problem. And we fully disclosed the professional mold test results to the buyer of our home. Again, not everyone has mold illness, and since I had reacted so strongly to that hotel room and our child's carseat, it was clear that my body was reacting to mold in a very unusual way. It was my body itself that had become too weak and broken down to deal with mold toxins.

At this time, I began reading about mold avoidance and discovered the phenomena of becoming "unmasked." The pieces began to fit together. It was a whirlwind of learning and coping, while sleeping on the floor at my parents house and selling all of our belongings. Though it was extremely traumatic and financially difficult, discovering mold in our home was actually exciting for me because it provided a clue about why I was still sick. Being healthy is, of course, much more important than houses and belongings. And I hadn't been getting better despite trying so many old treatments.

I am glad that I took an accidental mold sabbatical, because I'm not sure that I would have voluntarily done it, because I didn't suspect mold to be my issue.

Also during this time, I began "dumping," though I didn't know what dumping was at the time. Essentially, when the body is removed from mold toxicity, detox channels are turned back on, and the body starts releasing all kinds of junk that it had held onto tightly for years: mold toxins, heavy metals, and other biotoxins. This is why many people initially feel worse when they get out of mold while at the same time feeling better, which can be a very confusing experience. Interestingly, my body began to release more heavy metals than I had been able to get out in the past despite years of chelation therapies! It turns out that mold avoidance is actually the best heavy metal detox program.

And thus we became homeless. My wife and three kids bounced around friends and family's houses while I slept at my parents house; I didn't want to risk moving out of my parents' house at the time because it seemed safe to me and I didn't appear to be reacting to their house. My brain was also so affected still that I couldn't gather my thoughts enough to formulate a plan.

I began staying up late in the guest bedroom at my parents house and reading voraciously to determine what we should do next. There was, of course, the possibility of just moving into a different home in our city (South Lake Tahoe, CA). But the mold avoiders I spoke with and books I read, convinced me that it isn't just the indoor air which is responsible for making people sick, but can also be widespread outdoor air problems. I learned that Lake Tahoe is one of the greatest offenders for outdoor air issues, likely as a result of solvent spills decades ago which contaminated the sewer systems and caused the mold inside of them to begin making very strong mycotoxins, which we now loosely refer to as "Mystery Toxin" (or "MT"). Mystery Toxin was so-named because the illness which it causes has been a mystery to doctors, and because many people with this mystery illness do not realize they are being exposed to this toxin.

This particular toxin was so strong in Tahoe that some people even called it the "Tahoe Toxin." There was a whole list of strange outdoor toxins I had never heard about in the book, "The Beginner's Guide to Mold Avoidance."

During this time, I was experiencing a radical paradigm change in how I viewed healing from chronic disease. Most people with chronic disease are continuously *adding* things into their protocols. Adding supplements, antibiotics, vitamins and minerals, herbs, essential oils, rife treatments, hormones, and the list goes on and on. That particular approach hadn't seemed to work for me. And I gradually discovered that what my body really needed was instead to *take toxins away*, not add more treatments. This was a huge revelation! Later on in the healing process, my body would continue to become unmasked to many other toxins, including glyphosate, which experienced mold avoiders now believe has a detrimental effect on the body's healthy biome. I mean, I can actually now FEEL when I am exposed to glyphosate – it is not a philosophical disagreement with use of the chemical in our food supply. It is an actual reaction that tells me to stay away from it. The more I healed, the more I realized that my body wasn't missing important treatments, but instead, was being exposed to too many toxins. A paradigm change, indeed, compared to the days when all I wanted to do was to try new treatments.

Removing the mold part of the equation seemed to be a catalyst that allowed detox to occur, and all of a sudden I could feel a number of other toxins which were harming me, too; toxins which I hadn't noticed as bothersome when living in mold. For example, in addition to glyphosate, I began to be much more picky about the water I was drinking, and have my symptoms change a great deal depending on whether I was able to get my hands on drinking water that felt good to me. I was no longer able to eat non-organic foods. It seemed that taking mold out of the equation was finally allowing my body to communicate with me; to say, "please stay away from some of this stuff, it is killing you!" Before getting out of mold, the same poisons were probably still killing me, but I just couldn't feel it. Mold avoidance had not just unmasked me to mold, but also to many other things, in a perceptible and dramatic way. My body was yelling at me loudly, telling me what the problem was and why I was sick.

On the other hand, I had tried in years prior to remove these toxins, and that didn't work. Organic food and saunas and other toxin avoidance never helped. Mold was the "master toxin," the one which trumped all other toxins. It was as though the body was only willing to tackle the other toxins when the Big Daddy of toxins was first kicked out. And just as the experienced mold avoiders told me would happen, the more I avoided mold, the more I built up my resilience to be able to tolerate all of the "lesser toxins" once again. Multiple Chemical Sensitivity (MCS) just magically began to vanish after beginning mold avoidance, and food intolerances began to slowly melt away. I began to realize that the need for avoiding fragrances and chemicals was just a side effect of mold poisoning, and that these chemicals were trivial in comparison. Of course, all of our modern-world toxins really *are* bad for us, and we should make reasonable efforts to stay clear of them. But accidentally walking through a tiny cloud of perfume no longer affected me, and in fact, it smelled kind of nice!

So here I was, in the midst of these really overwhelming health discoveries, also trying to tackle the overwhelming problem of where our family should live. I remembered my RV dreams and after reading that many mold-sick people did well in RVs, I realized that this was our next step. It dawned on me that my RV fantasies were really my subconscious trying to send me a message. Well, message received, loud and clear! Since we were already moved out of our home and homeless, it wasn't a huge leap to imagine us in an RV. I read in *The Beginner's Guide* about a concept called "the locations effect," where mold-sick individuals noticed huge changes in their health depending on which locations they were exposed to. I figured that now was as good a time as ever to really dig in and test this concept. People who are this sick and finally discover such a big clue, become extremely motivated to find answers and get better. As Erik once famously said, "mold avoidance kicks ass." Now that I knew that, I wanted more of it!

At the time, I was feeling very worried because it wasn't just me, but my family of five, who seemed to be affected by the mold exposure. I was determined to find out if the entire Tahoe area was harming us. There would never be a better time to figure this out.

I began researching RV's and travel trailers. This intuitively felt like the right choice to me, to travel for the winter, avoid the winter time mold exacerbation, and learn about the locations effect. Little did I know at the time that these travels would unmask me even further and that we would make some huge, costly mistakes on the road; but mistakes which would serve to provide us an accelerated education on mold avoidance. And little did I know that I would return to Tahoe six months later, only to find that the entire region was too problematic for me to tolerate, at least at the time.

Of course, an RV or travel trailer is far from a perfect solution. These boxes on wheels are known for their toxicities; new ones contain a high level of formaldehyde and other chemicals, and old ones tend to be moldy. Thankfully, by this time, I was starting to clue in on the fact that mold is the master toxin, and so I was willing to put up with some lesser toxins in order to do mold avoidance. As Lisa and Erik have said, our modern society is very toxic in many ways, and avoiding ALL toxins is impossible. Attempting to do so will paralyze a person with indecision; thus, avoiding just the worst toxins should be the goal. So I figured that getting away from mold and being exposed to some chemicals was a good trade off. It turned out to be the right decision, as I continued to watch my chemical sensitivities vanish.

I made many trips to RV dealers to try to find an RV which was the least toxic feeling to me. I took a leap of faith, believing that whatever bad toxins we had escaped inside our home and city were making me much sicker than any new RV chemicals would. We settled on a 33-foot travel trailer and bought a new truck to pull it. We were able to find an RV brand which was environmentally conscious and used relatively non-toxic building materials.

I liked the idea of a separate truck and trailer rather than an RV where engine and living space are combined; this was the cheapest option, and it also made sense to me to have this extra flexibility where either component could be swapped out or mixed and matched as needed, especially if one unit became moldy and needed to be replaced. Furthermore, I discovered my 2002 4Runner (which I had bought new and owned for 15 years) was also riddled with mold toxicity, and I needed a new vehicle. A truck would serve as a new personal vehicle and a tow vehicle; whereas an RV would not offer this benefit and would force me to purchase two new motorized vehicles. The truck would also allow for the option of sleeping in the truck bed with a camper shell, which, as you'll see, turned out to be a life-saving amenity for me. You can read my "trailer buying tips for mold avoiders" here: www.lymebook.com/extreme-mold-avoidance

We frantically spent several weeks loading up the new travel trailer with freshly-purchased clothing and housewares, and getting ready to embark on our mold avoidance journey. It was the craziest time. We had to register the kids for a homeschool program and I had to train my employee on how to completely run my company while I was gone. All the while I was "dumping" toxins and trying to figure out what was happening to my body. The weather was changing and we were juggling rain and snow in a ski town. I had never owned or operated a diesel truck and travel trailer before. At the time I write this, I've now pulled our trailer more than 15,000 miles.

We were literally replacing or changing out of everything we owned, all in a 30 day period. Housing, vehicles, clothing, schooling, even location: all of these changed for our family in the blink of an eye. With no prior notice, and no help from insurance companies. This situation made a house fire seem like a cake walk, in comparison.

We set off on our journey on November 22, 2017. At the time, I really hadn't read enough yet about mold avoidance and I thought my only goals were to try out a lower elevation, be in a climate where we could be outdoors more often, and get away from any potential outdoor toxins in the

Tahoe basin. It turned out that I was on the right track, but as you will see, this was just the beginning. There was so much more to it than that. I was about as naive as can be when it came to mold avoidance.

The travels we had were very bitter-sweet, with very high highs and low lows. But looking back, the ozone ten pass treatments, the unintentional mold sabbatical, and the mold avoidance road trip definitely saved my life. Don't get me wrong, RV life for the purpose of mold avoidance is very challenging and there are various obstacles which people must confront. But getting your life back is a big accomplishment! Especially for people who are *really sick*, and for whom nothing is working anymore. Feeling better in that circumstance is nothing short of a miracle, and all the sacrifices are worth it.

I wrote this book while on the road, living in 200 square feet with my family of 5. Writing a book is hard enough when a person has quiet and privacy, so this was a real challenge!

Some parts of the book were written outdoors, in the sun, while sitting on boulders or logs. Or, in random buildings, usually Walmart, where the indoor air was tolerable to someone (me) who was in the "intensification" phase of mold illness healing. I've been writing for you about our experiences WHILE we are having these experiences.

I almost held off on writing this book until I could use my normal home-office tools to ensure the publishing and editing process went as smoothly as possible. But in the end, I chose to write the book amidst the chaos, to get the information to you sooner. So if the book seems a little rushed and not as polished as my other books, try to imagine what it is like to write a book in an RV with three kids!

Many people will be mad at me for writing this book, even if they don't realize they are mad. They will feel like I've challenged them to do something very difficult and even miserable: leaving one's home and belongings and restricting life by pursuing extreme mold avoidance. But remember,

I didn't write the rules. I'm just the messenger. I can no more change the truth of what is inside this book than I can stop the sun from rising. It is simply a fact that many people with horrible illnesses experience profound improvement when they pursue the kind of mold avoidance discussed in this book, even after all other treatments fail. This fact may not be one that you like, but nevertheless, facts are facts.

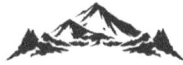

Chapter 8

DEFINING THE APPROACH

Now that you've had some introduction, I want to provide a few more details about how the approach described in this book differs from the normal mold toxicity protocols provided by most Lyme doctors and mold experts. Be it known that the approach in this book is VERY different from what you've heard from other sources.

I want to emphasize, though, that the information in this chapter is based on my own interpretation of the approach, and my own personal experiences. Lisa and Erik's books should be consulted directly to get the "official" details.

Essentially, the distinction is pretty simple. The approach in this book is based on the idea that extremely small amounts of mold and mold toxins can have a very powerful effect in keeping us sick, including outdoor mold toxins. And that the best way to find out which toxins are making us sick is not by running tests on our home or body, but instead, by getting really clear of mold toxins for a period of time so that our own bodies become unmasked and we are able to sense the toxins which make us most sick. We then use our own reactions to these toxins, instead of environmental mold tests, as a gauge for what we need to be avoiding, and for whether or not we are getting too much mold exposure in our air or environment. In essence, our bodies themselves become the test devices.

I believe that one of the reasons we fail to acknowledge the above principles is that we, as a society, are too emotionally attached to our homes and belongings to seriously entertain the possibility that they may be what is keeping us sick. And that even modern remediation techniques are still constrained by the desire people have to stay in their homes at all cost, and to not consider the possibility that their homes may be making them so sick that remediation won't solve the problem (at least for super-sick patients who have become extremely reactive to mold, not necessarily for the general population). In other words, the approach described in this book is never considered because we never want to consider it. The question is never asked, "is this approach valid." Instead, we ask the question, "is this approach something I want to believe."

One of the problems with mold is that it is a very "sticky" toxin, and once inside the body, is very hard to get out. It is also very hard to completely remove from living spaces. And it has also been observed that people with mold illness act as a magnet that attracts mold, which might also explain why such small amounts of mold can be a problem. (If you haven't noticed yet, mold is weird! Later in this book you'll find a chapter which discusses how important it is that we realize the weirdness of mold).

Since this is such a tough concept to fully grasp, let me approach it another way. If I asked you if you are completely well, what would you say?

I know with 100% certainty that you are not completely well. Why would I make such a brash, harsh statement? Because we live in a toxic world. Many types of toxins besiege us, including biotoxins (any toxin produced by a living organism such as mycotoxins, Lyme toxins, etc), heavy metals, electromagnetic fields (EMF's), and many other man made insults.

Chances are, you would answer my question by saying that no, you aren't completely well. You probably wouldn't be reading this book if you were. During our recoveries, most of us address as many of the toxic insults as we can. But over time, blindspots develop. We hyperfocus on eliminating certain contaminants (by eating organic food and not using toxic fragrances) but we completely ignore others.

As I mentioned, one of the reasons we ignore certain contaminants is because humans have developed a very peculiar behavior in comparison to other animals on planet Earth. This behavior is mainly driven by cultural norms and financial considerations. We have a strong, almost unchange-able desire to hold on tightly to our home, and our belongings. Which by definition includes our location, since our home is usually unmovable. Even when we do move, we usually bring all of our belongings with us. Of course, this behavior is understandable given our current cultural environment. Yet, if you look around the world, you will notice that animals don't normally do this. If an animal senses a life-threatening contamination or environmental threat in its environment, it will try to leave. But for humans, we just assume it is a given that we should be able to "fix" our home environment enough to be able to heal in it. But what if this assumption is wrong?

Many humans may have a deep inner intuition that leaving home or belongings is a good idea under some circumstances, but we rarely listen to that intuition because our cultural inputs are just too strong.

But by keeping all of our belongings and remaining in the same home (or even, sometimes, the same town) we are voluntarily submitting to one of the largest blind spots in the healing of any chronic disease: our environment.

And this is the crux of the difference between this book and "normal" approaches to mold treatment. Most mold therapies leave a person to still live in civilization and still be exposed to mold toxins, even if in small quantities. But the approach in this book acknowledges that it is sometimes necessary for people to get even more clear of mold toxins in order to kick-start healing. Much more clear than what most doctors would advise. And that in getting super-clear, the body's healing processes are jump-started, and that there is really no other way to achieve this success. In many cases, people experience incredible results from this approach even though they've already tried other mold therapies. The necessity of getting super-clear is typically not something that lasts forever. Eventually, most people are able to return to civilization. However, it is the initial super-clear phase of healing which is the most important, and which kick-starts the healing process. Kind of like how kids learn that rolling a snowball to a huge size is impossible if one doesn't start rolling it when it is much smaller in size.

Some people who have been extremely sick and debilitated, like myself, have decided they would do ANYTHING to get well, even leave all of their belongings, their home, and possibly even their city. Other people will decide that they are not willing to do this at all. And yet others will never even find out that this option exists.

New studies and schools of thought in the research world are rapidly identifying environmental toxins as the causes for many incurable diseases, including Parkinson's, Alzheimer's, and other forms of dementia and degenerative conditions. I didn't write these rules. I am simply sharing them.

Of course, not every person with mold sickness will need to pursue the same degree of mold avoidance in order to kick-start the healing process. Less sick folks will need less extreme measures. But what makes the approach in this book unique is that we are WILLING to do whatever it takes, and that our body is the one who tells us how much is necessary based on our reactions to mold. We realize that getting *clear enough* is what causes the body to basically wake from the dead and kick-start the detoxification processes which are supposed to be keeping these toxins at bay inside our bodies.

Before moving on, I want to spend a little more time talking about why very tiny amounts of mold toxins might be having such a profound effect on mold sick individuals. Erik Johnson was actually trained by the US Military to understand and implement decontamination procedures for extremely dangerous biological warfare agents, and he found that mold illness requires a very similar approach. What a paradigm change!

Lyme disease sufferers often end up with a condition called CIRS (Chronic Inflammatory Response Syndrome), also sometimes called Biotoxin Illness. This is, of course, old news. CIRS occurs when the body becomes flooded with biotoxins. Biotoxins are toxins from living organisms: mold, Lyme infections, and other organisms. Exposure to environmental mold AND internal infections can compound and accelerate the accumulation of bio-toxins inside the body, ushering in CIRS. And many researchers believe that CIRS patients are also colonized by mold internally, and so mold exposure can come from both inside and outside the body. When you are exposed to mold and also have Lyme disease, you have twice as many toxins.

Something interesting happens when the body fills up with toxins. If the exposure to those toxins – especially mycotoxins – continues, and is over-whelming to the body's defense systems, then the body sort of gives up on detoxing, and just starts to accumulate the toxins in tissues, especially fat stores and in the brain. This, of course, leads to continued worsening of disease. And this is where the approach in this book really diverges from normal mold detox approaches advocated by many doctors. Doctors often think that getting *relatively* clear of mold, and taking some detox supplements and drugs, will cause the body to adequately detox itself of mold. And while this may be true for many people, it is often *not* true of super-sick people. Why not?

Erik discovered something quite fascinating, which is still considered to be "rogue medicine" by many mold authorities. Erik found that the body simply will not engage in detox unless it is in a "safe location." That safe location is a place where the body is not being exposed to even small amounts of mold toxins. It sounds counter-intuitive – why would the body STOP detox-ing when it is needed most? But it has been consistently observed, and this single distinction makes ALL the difference. People who try to detox using the standard mold treatments often find themselves getting even sicker, if they aren't in a very clean location. By "location," I mean the air you breath, the shelter you live in, the clothes on your back, your bedding, and the level of mold on your skin. Even if the standard mold treatments help a little bit, it is working against the body, not with it.

The body isn't stupid. It is believed by those who understand Erik's approach that the body shuts down detox to protect itself from the ambient myco-toxins a person is being exposed to, and that the detox process is kind of a two-way street: if the body opens up to let mold out, it will also be letting mold in to the cells. I have personally experienced this numerous times, as have hundreds of other mold avoiders. When detox is turned on, the body is letting toxins in AND out of the cells. The body does not want to open up this two-way street unless it is certain that mold will not be coming in.

But there's more. In addition to shunting detox, being in a bad environment with even low levels of ambient mold also causes the body to lower oxygen flow to the tissues, which in and of itself is responsible for many of the symptoms of chronic illness. The lowered-oxygen state also encourages the growth and proliferation of all sorts of anaerobic chronic infections we talk about including Lyme, co-infections, parasites, and viruses. So there is a very high price to be paid for not being clear of mold toxins. And no matter how many supplements a person takes or what kinds of treatments they are doing, if the body doesn't decide it is safe to detox, progress will be severely limited. Thankfully, as recovery progresses, a person may be able to detox effectively in less and less "pristine" locations. But early on in the mold avoidance process, it is often necessary to kick-start the process by getting super-clear of mold toxins.

The body won't just stop detoxing mold toxins when you are living in a moldy environment. Detox also turns off for other toxins, including heavy metals. This is why some people notice that endless chelation and detox supplements seem to do nothing, or even make them worse. This happened to me while living in a moldy environment.

This is also why, when people initially get to a clean environment, they may feel worse even while they feel better, as the body turns detox back on, and years worth of toxins which were stored in the tissues come flooding out into the bloodstream. We are lucky to live in an era where this magnified detox phenomena has been identified. Before it was discovered, sometimes people actually confused good environments for bad environments because of the detox reaction. However, please note that when in a good location, people still feel MUCH better. Although the detox process can be uncomfortable, the relief and healing that comes from being free of these toxins far outweighs the detox symptoms.

The mold illness community, and one physician in particular who has mold illness himself and has been leading the charge in figuring this stuff out, has coined this intensive detox process with the term "dumping" (the process of dumping toxins during visits to really good, or "pristine," locations).

When I got out of mold, I experienced extreme dumping, but only when I visited locations with very good air and slept in shelters that were virtually mold free, including the back of my truck with an aluminum camper shell. I no longer need to do that in order to detox, but I had to do it in the beginning. I want to point out, though, that I felt MUCH better being out of mold. The "dumping" that was occuring in my body was only a minor nuisance compared to the overwhelming sense of relief and improvement that I felt. I don't want the dumping information here to discourage people from pursuing mold avoidance. Being away from the mold was the single most helpful thing I've ever done for my health.

The take-home point is that our bodies are either accumulating, or releasing, toxins. When living in mold exposure, it is just about impossible to recover from Lyme disease or any other chronic illness, because the body simply starts hoarding toxins and won't release them, even if you try to force it. In fact, many Lyme sufferers report that simply getting out of mold – and no other treatments – led them to more improvement than tens or hundreds of thousands of dollars in "treatments." The degree to which people need to get clear of mold depends on how sick they are. In some cases, regular mold treatments and simply leaving very moldy housing and moving into "decent" housing may be enough to recover. But for very sick people, the detox process may not be turned back on unless much more drastic measures are taken. This is why many people who follow Erik's approach only get better when they leave all of their contaminated belongings behind, and even live in RV's or tents for a period of time to allow the body to jumpstart the detox process. Remember, the body has been bombarded with these toxins for years or decades! It is unrealistic to expect that half-measures will do the trick.

Another aspect of Erik's approach is that being out of mold for a period of time actually results in mold reactions intensifying for a while. This is known as the "intensification" phase of healing, and is discussed in *The Beginner's Guide to Mold Avoidance*. This phase of healing is critical but is often overlooked by more standard mold approaches.

Most people are able to heal enough by doing continuing mold avoidance (as well as supportive therapies) that they can eventually begin to tolerate increasing levels of mold exposure without backsliding. Erik has named this process the "power curve," and staying high enough on the power curve will allow small mold exposures without dire consequences. But if too much mold exposure occurs, people can be knocked off the power curve and may need to struggle and do more extreme mold avoidance to climb back up the power curve. The place we want to be on the power curve is above the point, or threshold, where mold exposure shuts off detox and reactivates infections. Erik was even able to eventually go back to work in a moldy building, so long as he decontaminated before bedtime and slept in a very clear location, such as a metal cargo trailer in the woods. Again, not everyone will need to be this extreme, but some of the sickest people may need this.

And that brings us to the infectious component of mold illness. It has been observed that almost all mold-sick individuals have chronic infections and parasites. Almost all of them! Mold suppresses the immune system, turns off detox, reduces oxygen flow, and creates a perfect environment for infections to thrive. This is why getting out of mold is so important to heal.

I have personally also observed that even small mold exposures can cause reactivation of infections, and in my opinion, these small "mold hits" are actually directly interacting somehow with the infections in the body. Several researchers, including myself, have hypothesized that even very tiny levels of mold can directly aid the infections in their survival, possibly by acting as a building block for their biofilm. I'm also convinced that some mold exposures may act as communication, or quorum sensing, to wake up dormant infections in the body.

In other words, very SMALL mold exposures can have BIG conse-quences. Not just because of increased toxicity, but also because of a direct effect in awakening and supporting the survival of pathogenic microbes in the body.

So, is mold avoidance alone enough to heal people completely? I am not going to claim I have any answer to this question. Some people do manage to get much better with mold avoidance alone. Some get completely well. My observation is similar to what Lisa has told me, which is that mold avoidance alone is often not enough to heal people. But mold avoidance does allow the other issues a person is dealing with to be successfully dealt with, assuming the correct therapies are employed. Mold avoidance is a catalyst for pretty much any other therapy or healing methodology, even for diet and exercise. Mold avoidance is a leverage point, as Lisa says. Mold avoidance is the supercharge in the healing process.

What About a Less Extreme Version of Mold Avoidance?

A mentor of mine read my book before it was published and told me that I need to mention that not everyone needs to be as extreme as I am with mold avoidance. This is true. People who are less sick may be able to heal without taking quite as extreme measures.

My mentor told me that a lot of people will be turned off to mold avoidance if everyone thinks that the only way to do this is to be super extreme about it, and that it needs to be stated up front that not everyone needs to do this in the same way.

For example, my wife and children were not as sick as I was to start out, and they did not need to pursue mold avoidance at the same level that I have. This, of course, becomes a challenge for families. What if one family member has more extreme needs than the others? This is probably the most challenging aspect of doing mold avoidance with a family, and requires a lot of flexibility, learning from mistakes, compromises, understanding, and love. It also requires really carefully planning an ideal place to live, where both parties can get their needs met. For example, my ideal property purchase will be acreage that is about 30 minutes away from a city or town with good family resources. To basically have "one foot in each world." While I stay on the property and detox and hike, my family can go into town to participate in city activities. They can decontaminate upon coming back home, so we can all live together. I recently made a YouTube video which included this very topic; visit my YouTube channel entitled Lyme Disease Publisher, and watch the video called "Making Movements Toward Health."

So it is important to point out that this is an individualized process, which depends a lot on how sick a person starts out. There is no one-size-fits-all. And people should not be afraid to try mold avoidance, for fear that they cannot succeed in being as extreme as I have been. And if there is a family involved, careful thought and planning needs to be employed to make sure a proper balance is achieved.

I would like to talk more about the family aspects of mold avoidance in future books or videos, since this is an area where I believe there isn't a lot of adequate information.

Keep up with my future content by visiting: www.antilyme.com

Part II:

LESSONS
FROM THE ROAD

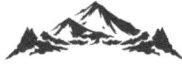

Chapter 9

OUR 25,000 MILE MOLD AVOIDANCE ROAD TRIP

The next several chapters of this book will be written as something of a travel diary, but I won't just be sharing our travel experiences like a normal travel journalist. I'll be sharing the mold avoidance lessons I learned at each stop along the way. Each destination has profound, practical lessons, which can be extracted for your own education and utility.

The approach described in this book has a very steep learning curve. In fact, many highly accomplished and intelligent people have said that doing this is the hardest thing they've ever done in their lives. Erik and Lisa have both said this, and I would say it too. Thankfully, Erik's discoveries and Lisa's effort in organizing them and adding her own research have made the learning process much more manageable. But still, the learning curve is steep and the sacrifices needed to achieve success are substantial. In addition to the two books co-authored by Erik and Lisa which I mentioned earlier (*The Beginner's Guide to Mold Avoidance* and *Back From The Edge*), it is now time for me to introduce you to their third book. *Erik On Avoidance* is the third book and much more of a technical, how-to guide for mold avoidance. I very much suggest that you read it at some point.

When I first joined the Mold Avoiders Facebook Group run by Lisa, I was surprised to see that many of the members were traveling around from place to place, as a part of their mold avoidance, often covering thousands of miles. While Erik himself didn't do this as much, I would later realize that travel has a number of benefits for mold avoiders, but more interestingly, I found out that a biological drive to travel through different areas, climates, and biomes seemed to actually be one of the symptoms of mold illness, especially once a person is able to leave their moldy environment and get clear. I could recall various times in my life, before I knew any of this stuff, when I made uncanny observations about how different locations affected how I felt. Healthy friends always just gave me a blank stare and say they'd never experienced anything like this.

There seems to be some biological, physiological need for a mold poisoned body to travel through different biomes and regions, perhaps to replenish the biodiversity inside the body by breathing and interacting with different microbes. It was almost as though my body knew that the balance of microorganisms living inside of me was toxic, and my body wanted me to go expose myself to new and different biomes, in order to help accumulate microbes from other environments, and repopulate the body-wide flora. Some have chalked up this travel desire to "fight or flight" syndrome, but I experienced it as something entirely different, and much more specific, than that. And, it may in fact turn out that this insatiable desire to move around was in fact driven by my body's own wisdom on how to heal itself. Perhaps my body was able to pick up new, healthier flora from the many environments we visited.

Some mold avoiders, including myself, noticed that this drive did dissipate as healing continued. I personally found that a strong urge to travel was actually one of the objective symptoms of mold toxicity. When first out of mold, I had a strong, almost obsessive, desire to move around from place to place. The desire was so intense and blinding that it almost consumed my entire identity. I've noticed that the same thing happens to many other mold avoiders; that is, that they "hit the road" and often cover thousands of miles in search of environments with less mold.

But even besides the apparent biological drive, a "mold avoidance road trip" is also known to have value in teaching people mold avoidance skills. When living in the same area, and traveling the same roads, and visiting the same buildings, it is very difficult to discern changes in how you feel from day to day as a result of various locations.

Let's say you have lived in the same city for 10 years. You would become so accustomed to that city that you'd grow numb and unaware of how the city affects you and even how different locations within the city affect you. People can become masked not only to the toxins in their home, but also the toxins in their town. That one co-infection you just can't shake – it may be active and unhindered due to a toxin you are exposed to in your local grocery store, but if you never experience that co-infection wax and wane due to changes in location, you would never figure out that location has an impact. Traveling and experiencing different climates, environments, and regions adds a level of clarity that you can't achieve any other way.

Usually, people don't experience this "locations effect" simply by taking their normal vacations and travels. Most people vacation and travel in the same locations over and over, for short periods of time, and often stay inside the same buildings. It is only by breaking free of these patterns that we can truly start to discover how locations may be affecting us. Also, most people vacation in very populated places and spend their time in conventional buildings. It definitely requires going off the beaten path to experience many of the very clear areas.

This is one of the major paradigm shifts required to understand the mold avoidance approach described in this book. Most people think of mold only as an indoor problem, something you get exposed to when living in a moldy home. But Erik and Lisa have discovered that many of the most damaging mold toxins actually exist outdoors, and can taint entire regions. And furthermore, even highly populated areas without these special out-door toxins can still have enough "regular" mold toxins in the outdoor air to prevent someone from getting clear enough of mold to really notice the locations effect. So, it is often necessary to experience more remote settings, away from manmade infrastructure, in order to experience the dramatic change in symptoms that can result from the locations effect. Super good locations where the air is very clear of mold toxins are often referred to by mold avoiders as "pristine locations."

I believe this is why my family has always loved tent camping, because unbeknownst to us, tent camping trips were the only times when we got really clear of civilization and mold exposures. I now know that one of our favorite tent camping spots also happens to be quite pristine. But without knowing exactly why we were experiencing healing there, it was quite unlikely for us to accidentally run into this effect in our normal lives. And so we always left camping trips having a really keen sense that something was taking place in our bodies, but never really understanding what it was about camping that caused this effect. We tried to guess what was going on, and came up with a number of hypotheses, but none of them turned out to be accurate.

In fact, sometimes I came home from camping trips and felt so good, only to be hammered by being back inside my house again, that I slept in a tent in the back yard to try to feel better. I figured maybe it was EMF from my house that was the problem, or lack of fresh air. I even considered the possibility of mold, but I quickly became re-masked and gave up on the inconvenience of sleeping outside.

And so traveling for mold avoidance makes a lot of sense. It can remove you from your normal routines, shopping habits, church, and city. Of course, embarking on a mold avoidance road trip is certainly not the only way to detox and learn mold avoidance skills. But my wife and I felt strongly that this is what God was calling us to do in November of 2017, even though we didn't fully understand all of this yet. I hope our experiences as shared in the subsequent chapters will help you in your own learning process, whether or not you ever personally travel for this purpose.

Our RV trip proceeded exactly as I had hoped. As we moved around to new places and stayed for extended durations, I experienced changes in symptoms which didn't budge in my home town and my home. It allowed me to say "ah ha, these symptoms really are connected to location." It blew me away, actually. I became such a believer in the locations effect that I now feel it is one of the primary drivers in chronic illness. There were a few times on the trip when I would feel extremely ill and sluggish, only to move to a new location and then all of a sudden feel consistently great and be able to hike for long distances. This experience has been shared by so many other mold avoiders that it has just become a given. Of course, people who don't suffer from mold illness won't experience this. This seems to be an experience that is limited to those whose bodies have been damaged by mold.

Also, these experiences and observations were not possible at all until I became unmasked, and until I purposely sought out "clear" locations instead of just traveling to places that sounded fun.

One thing is certain: Each and every day, humans continue to pollute and ruin our world, and give the bad molds more toxic food to eat. Experience and science has taught us that normal molds in nature do not make super-harmful toxins that cause people to have mold illness, but instead, it is the combination of mold and chemicals which produces the really harmful toxins. And this is why civilization, or "civilidevastation" as Erik calls it, is such a problem. And so if you do plan to travel to learn mold avoidance, it may be better to do so sooner than later, as the "good" locations continue to be harder and harder to find as they become more polluted with man made chemicals.

It also may be better to plan to travel off the beaten path, away from civilization. At first, this was very hard for me. I started out just staying close to bigger cities and attractions. It was hard to force myself to visit the more obscure, often less attractive places, where civilization hasn't yet taken hold.

Another reason that my family and other mold avoider families have traveled is to seek out a good place to settle, where the air is good, amenities are available nearby, and real estate prices are affordable.

Some people might wonder if all this fuss is worth it. Do we really need to be detectives and go to the grouble of identifying these sneaky mold toxins that we are normally masked to? Well, the answer is the same as the answer I always give to this question: it depends. For me personally, pursuing this approach was the only thing that gave me my life back, so it was definitely worth it. Is it worth it to you? How sick are you? These are questions only you can answer.

Personally, I was literally saying goodbye to my family, and so any years I get to remain on planet earth now feel like a bonus to me. And for that bonus ride, I really don't care where I live. I do care insomuch as it affects my family, but if I can feel good and heal somewhere, that is all the incentive I need. I now visit places which the old me would have scoffed at as ugly or undesirable, and I love and cherish these places where true, deep healing can be found and where I can feel my body desperately peel off layers of illness and increase in vitality. My whole definition of beauty has in fact morphed into something entirely different and new.

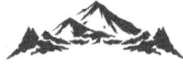

Chapter 10

SETTING OFF

After having sold, given away, or trashed just about everything we owned; purchasing a new truck and travel trailer, and hurriedly getting our affairs in order to leave, my family and I set off on the adventure – and challenge – of a lifetime. With the kids entered into an independent study program, and business affairs tidied up, we were as ready as we would ever be.

We initially tried to stay in dry, warm areas. We started off in Tonopah, NV, then spent a week at Oasis RV Resort in Las Vegas. It was still early in our trip, and we hadn't yet learned that we would fare better if we stayed further away from civilization (or, as Erik calls it, "civilidevastation"). We were beginner mold avoiders. I called it "mold avoidance kindergarten." I laughably thought that "mold avoidance" simply meant staying where it is warm.

After Las Vegas, we went to Oceanside, CA and stayed at an RV park in Vista, CA, for 3 weeks, which allowed me to do more 10 pass ozone with Dr. Shannon (you'll be reading more about this soon).

At this point, we thought we were doing enough mold avoidance. We weren't aware of the "dumping" phenomenon yet. And we hadn't had our first "mold hit" after being unmasked, yet. So it was all quite innocent and fun. We would later learn that being unmasked doesn't just happen in one singular event; it can happen in layers, and the longer you stay away from the toxins in civilization, the more your body becomes aware of them and the more your body tells you to avoid them.

Although we stayed in more than 50 places during our road trip, I am going to focus on and write about only the stops during which we learned the most.

Also, I would later learn that this "road trip" wasn't so much a singular occurrence, but that it was actually a new way of life. As I write this 15 months after setting out on the road, we are still living in our RV and healing. We've made incredible progress and are very happy with our choices. Most of the supplements and treatments that used to be "mandatory" for me to remain stable, and which I diligently packed into the storage compartment of our RV, now sit untouched and forgotten, due to the unimaginable health improvements I've experienced while doing mold avoidance.

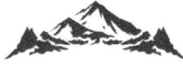

Chapter 11

SAN DIEGO, CA

After leaving Oceanside, I intuitively knew I needed to go to the desert. In fact, back when I first got out of our mold house, I was actually waking up in the middle of the night having visions and dreams of the desert!

But before we went to the desert, we thought we'd make one last "fun stop" in San Diego (near Chula Vista, to be exact). We wanted to take the kids to the zoo, and all the other great attractions in San Diego.

But, looking back now with more experience, I can see something else was motivating me. The process of detoxing, or dumping, can be somewhat uncomfortable, and I think I was starting to detox. I think I was resistant to going to the desert because intuitively I knew it would accelerate the detox process. So I steered us to San Diego, and not to the desert. Later I would learn that turning off the detox response by going into less-than-pristine areas can actually lead to a temporary relief in symptoms. Of course, in the long run, one does need to seek and begin the detox process, in order to lower the toxin load. Also, I would later learn that one of the reasons for discomfort while detoxing is that many people force-feed themselves a wide variety of binders and supplements during detox. It has been observed by many mold avoiders that simply letting the body naturally heal itself in pristine locations leads to faster improvement and less discomfort than occurs when detox supplements are used. Lisa probably said it best when she stated that detox supplements should only be used if they make you feel better, not worse. I've come to agree with her on this.

Anyway, Chula Vista turned out to be a far different experience than what we had banked on. We stayed at an RV resort close to the San Diego bay. The trouble that would befall us at Chula Vista would cost us over $10,000 and almost two months of difficulty. Still, though, looking back, I believe that the Chula Vista catastrophe was a blessing in disguise, because it forced us to up the ante in our mold avoidance education. It was the push we needed to take things to the next level, do more reading, and continue on the path to healing.

Chula Vista – those two words – have become dark, dark words in our family. Probably like "Vietnam" is a powerful, emotional, and traumatic term for many Vets.

We only stayed near Chula Vista for one night. Yes, one night. You are probably wondering how such a bad thing could happen in one night, right?

As we've discussed, many of the worst mold toxins keeping people sick are not the ones found inside bad houses, but instead, outdoor mold toxins, and outdoor mold "plumes." Of course, we didn't know that at the time. Nor had we yet read about the conditions which create the worst outdoor molds; namely, the combination of living mold with manmade toxic chemicals.

It turns out that Chula Vista is one of many areas in the United States which is known for bad outdoor mold toxins. Many conditions converged there to create the perfect environment for outdoor supertoxins to be pro-duced in great quantity (you'll read about supertoxins in *The Beginner's Guide*). The area where we stayed was just a few blocks away from a famous industrial dump site that contained dozens of known highly toxic contaminants, which apparently caused a very bad kind of mold to grow and release outdoor toxins. Of course, it doesn't help that the whole San Diego bay is stagnant or that Mexico is known to dump millions of gallons of sewage into the nearby ocean. Sewage is also associated with the production of mold supertoxins.

While Chula Vista isn't that much different from many other "bad zones" around the country, I think our experience there was particularly hard due to the fact that we were in that "intensification" phase of healing, where all of our reactivities were heightened. Many people notice that certain early mold exposures after being unmasked have particularly damaging results, due to the increased reactivity that occurs during this phase of healing. Some people can later return to these same spots with a much smaller reaction, as their body moves out of intensification.

Right when we arrived at this RV park in San Diego, near Chula Vista, I began having very strange symptoms. A strong feeling of depression and doom. A weird kind of brain fog which was more extreme yet different from any other brain fog I had felt. Because I hadn't yet read *The Beginner's Guide,* I didn't know that these were telltale warning signs for a bad outdoor supertoxin, and that the appropriate course of action would have been to hook up the trailer, and get out of there at top speed.

I didn't know those details. So we stayed. At about 11pm, I woke up gasping for air, shuddering and shaking, and feeling the exact same symptoms that I felt that night in my home when I was first unmasked. It was terrible and crazy, and the first time we had encountered bad mold since leaving Tahoe.

We should have woken up in the middle of the night and left. Why? Not because of my health; that could have waited until the morning. What we didn't know was that these outdoor mold plumes are capable of inflicting severe and long-term contamination upon vehicles, property, and RVs. We didn't realize we were becoming badly contaminated, and because our immune systems had been out of mold and were healing, we wouldn't be able to tolerate being inside the RV after we left Chula Vista. We were ignorant.

We woke up in the morning and knew we had to leave, but took our time. The doom and strange symptoms were still in the air. We hooked up, and drove to Yuma, AZ, our first desert stop. We took the kids to a few cool tourist destinations. We didn't yet realize the contamination we had picked up. It took our bodies a few days to start reacting to the contamination.

In mold avoidance, contamination picked up on your body, clothing, or belongings from an incident like this is known as "cross-contamination." That is, contamination which results not from primary mold growth on your belongings, but instead, from being exposed to a moldy environment and leaving that environment with mold toxins on your body, clothing, and belongings.

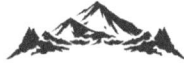

Chapter 12

TUCSON, AZ

When we were still in Tahoe, I just foolishly assumed that anywhere in the Southwest would be pristine desert. The visions I used to get of the desert were very nondescript. I figured that anywhere with cacti and dryness and a scorching sun would be healing to my body and mind and spirit.

I was wrong. Tucson turned out to be a huge mix of bad outdoor toxins, industrial pollution, and other issues. In his writings, Erik referred to the GFD, or God Forsaken Desert. But I would later learn from speaking with him, and from my own experiences, that what this really means is getting far away from civilization, and not necessarily just to the desert. Any climate, no matter how humid or dry, could qualify as the GFD and could be a healing place, as long as it was untainted by "civilidevastation." Which, specifically, means electromagnetic pollution, chemicals, manmade structures, sewer systems, vehicle exhaust, and other related marvels of society.

These tainted features of civilization are not in and of themselves what cause mold sick people to be harmed. Instead, these features have the potential to damage the natural biome and cause the local molds to produce harmful mold toxins. This is a very important distinction. I would later notice that such things as pollution and car exhaust had very little negative impact on me, unless mold was also present in a location. This distinction is critical and is where many people go wrong. Many people try to avoid ALL toxins, as if they are all created equal. This is such a difficult concept to un-learn, because it requires un-learning everything we are taught about being healthy. We are taught that pretty much all pollution and chemicals are bad for us. But what Erik found, and my experiences agree, is that once mold exposure is removed, the body heals itself and has a remarkable resilience when faced with these lesser toxins. In fact, mold turns out to be the "master toxin" which controls a person's reactivity to the other toxins and pollutants, at least for people with this sort of illness.

A very well-respected and brilliant mercury poisoning expert once told me that mercury was the master toxin, and the extent to which someone was mercury poisoned determined the level of reactivity they would have to other toxins. Yet, my experience was just the opposite. My mercury issues were easily and swiftly brought under control when mold toxicity was addressed.

A similar observation can be made with regard to fire retardant chemicals. Many mold-sick people notice that forest fire zones where fire retardants have been used cause mold illness to become much worse. But the interesting thing is that the chemicals themselves are not at all the problem; when exposed to just the chemicals, sickness does not result. Instead, the chemicals alter the biome and cause local mold to produce very harmful toxins which are responsible for doing the health damage.

Of course, this is not to say that pollution and fire retardant chemicals are safe. Of course they are not safe and are bad for us! There's no question about that. But for mold-sick people, the mold toxins produced in areas where pollution and fire retardants are present are a much bigger factor than the chemicals themselves. If I had to guess, I would say the mold toxins are 1,000 times more damaging than the chemicals themselves, in the context of mold illness.

But, let's get back to Tucson.

After Yuma, we rolled into Tucson and stayed at a nice RV park at the recommendation of another mold avoider who was residing there. It was at this time that we started to feel horrible reactions when spending time inside our travel trailer. I couldn't even be inside for more than 5 minutes. I would begin to have debilitating mold reactions that were very similar to how I felt in my old home, and I would experience extreme immuno-suppression that would reactivate old Lyme infections. Interestingly, this couldn't have even been the placebo effect, because at the time, I hadn't even yet learned about what is known as "cross contamination" (when a bad location or item can contaminate your space). So I didn't yet know we had picked up that much mold from the San Diego / Chula Vista stay.

We were in denial for a couple weeks. We didn't know just how bad the situation was. We ended up wasting a lot of money on useless efforts to remediate the RV. My new truck was also affected, so the situation was serious! We even ripped out the carpets from our brand new travel trailer and Dodge Ram. We were ripping apart our brand new property. That is how reactive we were. Within 6 weeks of their purchase, I had placed both RV and truck up for sale on Craig's List. Crazy, right? And this was just one night in Chula Vista.

You see, that mold in the air in Chula Vista had gotten inside our truck and trailer and contaminated them. As you may know, mold is comprised of mold spores. Think of these spores as little hard-shelled, pea-shaped spheres, filled with mycotoxins. The mycotoxins themselves are VOCs, that is, volatile organic compounds, just like perfume and paint fumes. If you are in the path of an outdoor mold plume but are relatively far away from the sourcepoint, you may be lucky and only pick up some of the VOCs. But if you are close enough to a source point, as we apparently were in Chula Vista, you may actually pick up spores themselves on your belongings. While there is some risk that these spores could be viable and could start a mold infestation in your possessions, the more certain danger is that once inside your property, these mold spores will start to continuously release their mycotoxins, on an going basis, for weeks or months. Like a hot air balloon leaking its contents. Certain conditions can accelerate or slow the release. Once released, these nasty mycotoxins tend to float around through the air and be absorbed into porous surfaces, and also tend to bond tightly with plastics and synthetic materials, thus turning all of our manmade, chemical-laden trailer and truck surfaces into mold-saturated sources of super badness. Because we picked up actual spores, and not just their VOCs, the release of toxins was ongoing and despite ripping out carpets, and vacuuming over and over, and wiping everything down, our efforts seemed to be in vain.

It was at this point that we realized that I myself was not the only one in our family affected by mold. It appeared that all five of us, to varying degrees, were reacting to Chula Vista badness. We were ALL now more sensitive to mold after having been out of our mold house, a well described process that occurs during the healing process, and is known as "intensification." The fact that the family was very affected by objective physical symptoms, also helped me to realize that I wasn't just insane and delusional about all of this (because I was starting to wonder!). My daughter quickly developed pale, blotchy skin and swollen eyes, my wife began getting headaches inside the trailer, and the other family members also saw symptoms that we hadn't felt since Tahoe. My son would eventually get sick from mold exposures as well, including aches, fever, and fatigue.

Fortunately, at the advice of other mold avoiders, I had purchased a metal camper shell for my truck (I started with a fiberglass shell, but the fiberglass offgassing was too strong and I swapped it out for a metal one). Since I was more affected than my family, they continued to sleep in the trailer while I slept in the back of the truck with electric space heaters. But we had no idea what to do next. We were stuck in a constant daily struggle to just survive, and the kids and my wife were becoming increasingly sick from the contamination in the trailer. Remember that before the Chula Vista event, we were all fine in the trailer. It was a one night contamination event which did this to us.

At this point, I did question whether this whole ordeal was even worth it. Maybe we should just forget about this, and go get a hotel, or rent a house. However, by this time I also began to notice some miraculous improvements in my health. So even though my body was telling me to avoid mold in tiny quantities, if I listened to my body and actually did my best to comply, I found that the payoff was worth it! Getting my life back was no small achievement.

We came to the decision as a family that my wife and kids would fly to Texas to stay with my wife's parents (the kids' grandparents) for a week or two while I stayed behind to figure out what to do. At this point, we were literally homeless. Our house in Tahoe was rented out, and our trailer was unlivable. While my family was in Texas, I was living in the back of my truck. I tried a few hotels, but due to being in "intensification," I couldn't tolerate them due to various levels of mold. It felt very strange to be homeless yet surrounded by homes and hotels. It wasn't lack money that was keeping me homeless (though we were also financially strained from this), it was lack of housing. As it turns out, housing is the single biggest challenge for people living with this illness.

While my family was gone, I began reading Erik and Lisa's books voraciously and consulting the many very knowledgeable people on the mold avoiders forum. It was suggested to me that bringing the truck and trailer to high elevation and cleaning them there would be helpful. I tried this several times by making the trek up to 8,000 feet, to the top of Mt. Lemmon. I definitely noticed that the toxins were more perceptible at high elevation; this was also the experience of others. They seemed to be less sticky and release more easily up there. One of Erik's discoveries was that mold spores released their toxins upon barometric pressure drops, which occur before storms but also occur as one travels up in elevation.

Mostly during this time, I was just in stunned disbelief. So much money in new truck and trailer, and our only home, was unlivable. But something else was going on. I was beginning to suspect that I was experiencing symptoms from outdoor mold toxins in Tucson. It seemed so crazy. Could these toxins really be affecting me while thousands of other people go about their days unaffected? This is why it was so important to go out on the road; these subtle observations would not be believable unless they were experienced numerous times in varying locations. Sure enough, many mold avoiders told me that Tucson was a known bad area for outdoor supertoxins. I began to match up my symptoms with super toxins described in Lisa and Erik's books. So now, I was dealing with two sets of toxins; those I picked up inside my truck and trailer, and those which were in the outdoor air in Tucson. But, I was told, this was all part of the learning process in discovering how to successfully be a mold avoider and recover.

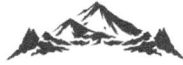

Chapter 13

SILVER CITY, NM

After languishing in Tucson for at least a couple of weeks in indecision and toxin symptoms, an experienced mold avoider convinced me that I wouldn't be able to make sense of the truck and trailer until I got out of Tucson and got to "good air." Thankfully, this person convinced me to pull my truck and trailer off of Craigslist until I had a better handle on things. While being exposed to the outdoor air in Tucson, I was told, I wouldn't be able to think clearly and to evaluate the truck and trailer. Also, in clean air, a person can spend the day (or longer) away from their property to "get clear," and then return to the items to see how they feel.

This was the first time I really read about the "good air" concept; that is, that the toxin dumping and detox process won't start until a person gets to good air, and also, that one won't really be able to make sense of their belongings until the air itself isn't confusing the issue.

It turns out that many new mold avoiders have a hard time getting to good air. Why? Because all of our lives, we are taught that we should go to beautiful, popular areas for vacation. Big cities also have stores, activities, amenities, and attractions. Getting to clean air often requires going way off of the beaten path, to places where normal people don't want to go. Of course, many of us were brought up camping and backpacking, so that kind of background definitely helps.

Another thing I was learning was that how a place looks isn't a good predictor of how good the air is. A beautiful outdoorsy setting may have bad air. And some larger cities have good air. It is very hard to predict. This is why it is so important to become unmasked, so you can feel *for yourself* where the air is good, and which buildings are safe. I rarely, if ever, hear about people making good recoveries when they are solely relying on laboratory testing rather than their own senses.

So I left Tucson and headed East into New Mexico in search of "good air." I had heard that Silver City, NM, was a relatively good-air destination. At this point, my family remained with the in-laws in Texas.

On the way to Silver City, I spent the night in Lordsburg, NM. it was such a strange experience, sleeping in the back of my truck at a KOA, 33 foot trailer hooked up but uninhabitable, my family gone, in a strange city and state I have never been in. Words barely describe it.

But something amazing and unbelievable happened. Lordsburg had very clear air at the time. I began to feel all of the areas in my body that had previously been affected by Lyme disease and mold. Everything started going nuts. It was very uncomfortable but intuitively felt like a healing process. I even began tasting and choking up what felt very much like agricultural toxins. At first, I was sure that the KOA itself was contaminated and the source of the agricultural toxins. But I soon realized that these toxins were coming out of ME, not the environment. Other areas of my body where I've had infections and issues started hurting and throbbing and swelling. Could this all have been happening just because of the clean air? Was that really possible? Everyone told me it was possible. The clean air was a signal to my body to detox, and so I finally began heal from years of living in bad environments. The clean air literally acts like a sponge, via osmosis, where toxins are traveling from areas of higher concentration (my body) to areas of low concentration (the outdoor air). Toxins were being sucked out of my body.

After one night in Lordsburg, I continued up to Silver City. I still didn't have a plan to reunite with my family or any idea of what home we would live in, or if the truck and trailer were fixable. But I took the advice of other mold avoiders and decided to face these questions in "good air." And I'm glad I did, because things became much more clear.

But before I continue, I need to share just how much I started detoxing. I had so many mycotoxins coming out of me (due to the body sensing the good environment and releasing toxins) that I felt like I was on psychedelic drugs. Silver City seemed like this crazy, magical place to me, and all the sights and sounds took on a stranger, alternate reality experience. I know this wasn't silver city itself, because I would later visit the city again when the toxin "dumping" was not happening, and it was just a normal city, nothing magical about it.

The psychedelic feelings were so strong, that they completely took over my mind. I became convinced that Silver City was somehow the only place I could heal, and I planned and plotted our move there. I schemed and searched for rental houses, a church, and community involvement. Later, of course, I would realize that I was under the severe influence of mycotoxin dumping and detox. It turns out that some mycotoxins do in fact have a similar molecular structure as psychedelic drugs, which explains my experience.

Also during this time, my body didn't just start dumping mycotoxins. It started dumping heavy metals to an extent I couldn't' even believe. I had previously done hundreds, if not thousands of days of frequent-dose chelation as described by Andrew Cutler, and yet in just a few weeks in Silver City, I had more metals come out of me than years of chelation combined. It was all I could do to try to keep up with the waterfall of toxins coming out of my body; gobbling binders and chelators as fast as I could to stay ahead of the tidal wave that was coming out of me.

(I would like to note that some mold avoiders believe that it is best not to take binders and supplements during this phase of detox, and that doing so can make the detox process much more uncomfortable and even harmful. In fact, Lisa recommends that people not push detox at all, and just let the body naturally process and heal when clear of mold. I hadn't yet read that recommendation during this time, and so I might have saved myself a bit of discomfort with that information. One thing Lisa has always said is that if any particular detox supplement or therapy makes you feel worse, then you shouldn't use it.)

The doctor I mentioned earlier who himself has dealt with mold illness and who pioneered much of this information, told me to expect signs and symptoms of major heavy metal detox which included increased bile production, liver pain, neurological and blood circulation heavy metal symptoms, and more. And it all happened just as he said it would. It was very helpful that I was sleeping in the back of a metal truck bed, and staying in good air. These two factors were what allowed my body to detox, for the first time in years or decades (except for our tent camping trips).

Still, even while detoxing, I was beginning to feel the best I had felt in years. The discomfort of detoxing was far outweighed by the relief and improved health that I was beginning to feel. In fact, it was becoming ever more apparent that this mold avoidance thing was the missing puzzle piece in my healing.

The trailer continued to be uninhabitable in Silver City. The truck as well. I was able to remediate the bed of the truck and my metal camper shell because that space was just smooth metal. But the cab of the truck, with all of the leather and plastic and fabric, just wasn't improving enough.

By this time, my family had had enough of staying with the In-laws in Texas and they needed to move on. Since we could not live in the trailer, I decided to rent an Airbnb. I was also advised by mold avoiders to rent a car, so that while we were staying at the Airbnb we could spend some time away from all of our possessions and then come back to them at a later date in order to assess how they affected us.

It's funny; during our road trip I ended up driving back and forth between Silver City and Tucson many times; I don't remember exactly how many, but it was at least four. We put over 12,000 miles on the new truck in a four month period traveling only in the Southwest. We spent a MASSIVE amount of time and energy driving back and forth to and from various places, during different weather conditions, to accomplish different tasks of mold avoidance. This gave me a huge amount of experience with different places and how they compared to Tahoe, and how things like weather, elevation, and wind affected outdoor air quality.

One such drive from Silver City back to Tucson was to go fetch my family from the Tucson airport. Later that night we arrived at the Airbnb. Although we enjoyed staying there for about 4 days, there was a huge amount of stress and tension in the air because we literally had nowhere to go after our reservation concluded. Literally, nowhere to go. and now we were paying for a truck, a trailer, a rental car, and an expensive Airbnb. it was such insanity.

And things were about to get even more complicated. Little did we know, we were being contaminated again. The Airbnb we were staying at was badly saturated with a different mold toxin, a supertoxin which is sometimes referred to as HCCT (Highly Cross-Contaminating Toxin). This toxin has also previously been called "Hell Toxin," and it is described in *A Beginner's Guide to Mold Avoidance*. Science has yet to officially study and identify this toxin, and the name "Hell Toxin" is just a nickname that mold avoiders have given the toxin because one of its initial symptoms is typically itching and burning. At some point, hopefully science will be able to provide a more descriptive term for it. But it seems to be a relatively new toxin, and so much is still unknown.

I know, I know. It sounds like fiction. I didn't believe this stuff either, until it happened to me. One of the problems, I think, is that these toxins haven't been identified yet by science, and so they seem like mysterious, magical substances. In reality though, science has confirmed that mycotoxins cause damage to the human body in dozens of different ways. We just don't know which particular mycotoxin this is, yet.

Of course, being in the intensification phase of healing, we were extremely sensitive to mold toxins and every time we ran into them, it felt like it was catastrophic. Many people advised us not to make big life decisions when in intensification, because the health situation changes so rapidly and drastically from day to day and week to week. You don't want to thrash about and spend all of your money. "Conserve financial resources," one mold avoider told me.

Being beginner mold avoiders, we were foolish and brought just about everything we owned into that Airbnb. So, it all got contaminated. We had to throw it all away. We left the Airbnb surrounded by even more chaos than when we arrived. We went to a hotel room, which also turned out to be moldy. Our trailer was parked at a nearby RV park where they were starting to wonder why there was an RV parked there but no people, so we were about to get kicked out of there, too. Everything just seemed to keep going from bad to worse. But, as my wife wisely kept pointing out, it was all a learning experience that would benefit us later.

The toxin we've nicknamed "Hell Toxin" is unique. It doesn't behave like other mycotoxins. It seems to have some magnetic qualities to it, and is attracted to heavy metals. People with heavy metal poisoning have a much harder time and more extreme symptoms when exposed to hell toxin, and the toxin seems to literally be attracted to people and objects with a lot of metal in them, including electronics, computers, smartphones, and related items.

If you think this sounds crazy, go read about mold in the scientific literature. Some mold has actually been found to use and process heavy metals as food, and other mold has been found to be able to grow INSIDE nuclear powerplants where no other life can survive. It even grows faster when it consumes radioactivity; the radioactivity acts like food and fertilizer. Mold is a very strange organism and once you start reading about it, you realize that it behaves differently than just about any other living thing on the planet.

In the hotel room, my wife and I carefully analyzed our options. Our truck and trailer were still uninhabitable due to the Chula Vista incident. Should we sell the truck and trailer? Should we trade in the trailer for a new one? Where would we live? When I originally purchased the trailer, one of the attractive aspects of trailer life was how much cheaper it is to swap out a trailer than a house. Because our trailer was a current year model, the trade in loss would be relatively minimal. I never ACTUALLY thought we would end up trading in the trailer for a new one, though. It just seemed so sci-fi. But, here we were.

After much debate and discussion, we decided we wanted to start over and trade in the trailer for a new one. We picked the exact same brand and model since we already knew the ins-and-outs of using it and since we did not react badly to the chemicals they use to build it. You have to understand just how insane our friends thought we were. Trading in a brand new trailer because of some mysterious contamination that it picked up in one night, yes only one night, at an RV park where everyone else was happily enjoying their RV vacation. Only the dozens, even hundreds of similar stories on the mold avoider forum provided the confirmation that we needed that this type of thing can in fact happen to people with biotoxin illness.

We decided to keep the truck. The truck would be much more expensive to trade in, and a clean inside space in a vehicle was much less important than the living space where we sleep and spend all of our time. The con-tamination in the truck did eventually calm down, a few months later, by the way. While the trailer may have calmed down too, eventually, we didn't have time to wait for that to happen.

I located a new trailer at a dealership Arizona. While I went to go complete the trade and pick it up, my family stayed at a nice hotel in Tucson which, as far as we could tell, was only slightly affected by mold.

I came back to Tucson to park the new trailer at the hotel where the family was staying. But I started feeling symptoms of the same outdoor toxin I had felt in the RV park several weeks prior in Tucson. Now I was really panicking: could I be contaminating our new trailer, AGAIN? Why the heck was I back in Tucson, anyway? Hadn't I learned my lesson? At midnight, I made the decision to just leave Tucson. Just drive away, with truck and 33 foot trailer attached, into the night, with no idea where I would end up. I just had to get away, to prevent the contamination from happening again. I drove from midnight to 1am and ended up in Benson, AZ, sleeping half the night at a truck stop and the other half in a Walmart parking lot. My wife still had the rental car, so when she woke up in the morning at the hotel, she drove to Benson and met me at the local Walmart where we spent at least $1,500 restocking the trailer and replacing items that were contaminated with Hell Toxin from the Airbnb, or with the Chula Vista toxins (yes, now we were replacing items from TWO contamination events).

After restocking the trailer and staying one night in a horrible RV Park in Benson, and making a day trip to tour some amazing local caverns and the old cowboy town of Tombstone, AZ, we were looking for a place to land. We really wanted to be at an RV park with good air, and which could serve as a healing place for us after all we had been through. But now with a new trailer in tow and new belongings, I was becoming increasingly aware of the possibility of picking the wrong locations and ending up with further contamination. It became quite stressful to try to pick RV parks. We found we did best camping for free in public BLM land (Bureau of Land Management), or at national or state parks. But we couldn't simply camp out in the woods forever, because we needed RV hookups; we needed water, power, and sewer hookups to do laundry in our portable washer/dryer, to wash dishes, and to recharge the battery in the trailer. But I was certainly finding the whole idea of "civilidevastation" to be a real thing!

We were also beginning to discover, as other mold avoiders had discovered, that sewer systems tended to be the major sources of bad mold toxins; especially sewer sources that were near manmade chemical residue. Unfortunately, many sewer systems at RV parks ended up being very harmful to us and very toxic, due to bad kinds of mold growing in the sewer systems.

We were all exhausted, scared, and financially traumatized. We were starting to question whether a new trailer had been the right choice. We just couldn't seem to imagine finding a perfect RV park where the setting was healing and serene, where the kids could play and do homeschool, where the air was good, and where the sewer system wasn't harming us. It just seemed like an impossible feat; it seemed so unlikely. It was funny; at this point in the trip, we had been on the road for over two months but still hadn't been able to enjoy a good air location in a non-contaminated trailer. We had been on the road for two months and while we had learned a lot, we still hadn't had much opportunity to detox in peace and quiet and enjoy the healing benefits of the desert.

But, such a magical, healing place, is just what God would bring to us. Little did we know, we were about to discover the best, most healing destination of our entire trip. A place where we would experience much peace and happiness, learn a great deal, and finally get on with the business of detoxing and learning mold avoidance.

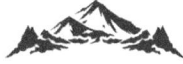

Chapter 14

DRAGOON, AZ

Dragoon wasn't just a stop on our trip. It started out that way. But it ended up being much more. It wasn't just a good RV park. It saved us. It redeemed our road trip. It bridged the gap between the first half of our trip (characterized by strife, mistakes, financial devastation, and desperation) and the last half of our trip (characterized by healing, detoxing, learning, and yes, some manageable challenges and struggles).

Without Dragoon, I'm not sure we would have been successful at mold avoidance. I'm not sure we would have healed enough, learned enough, or even been able to continue. I would have probably ended up just giving up on the whole thing.

My wife found the magical RV park in Dragoon on an RV park app on her phone. I had missed it and was about to just drive right by. She found it and insisted we go check it out. We literally exited the freeway at the last minute, as it was getting dark, with nowhere else to even go.

The place we stayed in Dragoon is a 160 acre "guest ranch" with cabins, horses, and lots of land. The kids got horseback riding lessons and got to run around in a safe place. The property contains huge, even gargantuan, boulders strewn about. We have found that massive boulders nearby seem to aid in the recovery process; exactly how, we aren't sure. The owner of the property was extremely kind to us, and the RV park portion where we stayed was magical and beautiful.

But most importantly, we had about 4 weeks of peaceful time in this place in good air. My detox continued and intensified. Metals and mold toxins were flowing out of my like a waterfall. I continued to sleep in the back of the truck, to maximize my exposure to fresh air and minimize any indoor pollutants I would be exposed to in the trailer, even though it was new. I would later learn that even sleeping near family members who are detoxing can be undesirable, and later I would endeavor to sleep separately from my family so that the toxins they were detoxing during their own breathing wouldn't contaminate my air. Thankfully, this became less and less necessary the more I healed.

It was during this time that I began to experience firsthand many of the nuances of mold avoidance that I read about in *The Beginner's Guide to Mold Avoidance* and in *Erik on Avoidance*. For example, taking frequent showers would provide intense and immediate symptom relief; presumably because washing off the mold toxins that came out of my pores renewed the "clean" environment my body needed to keep detoxing. I also noticed that brand new tshirts purchased from Walmart and washed and which had no perceptible odor, began to reek of mold after I wore them for only half a day. I was literally dumping mold toxins out of my pores. Intense and inexplicable excessive thirst and frequent urination I had had for close to two decades, just started to disappear. All of my stools (sorry, I don't want to be gross, but this is important) were coated in bile; a sign that the body is finally turning on bile flow. Bile is the single most important shuttle for fat soluble toxins to exit the body. Many chelators and supplements which I normally couldn't tolerate, became tolerable to me (this is also noticed by many other mold avoiders; that detox supplements are intolerable when living in mold because the body is fighting, not aiding, the detox process).

I learned that mold avoidance is just as much an intimate affair as it is an issue of the outdoor air. It is extremely important to especially avoid any mold when it comes to what is actually in contact with the body. This means that clothing and bedding plays a particularly important role in mold avoidance; that is, keeping them free of mold and mold cross-contamination.

Mold on the skin can quickly and violently shut down detox, and so frequent showers in good water become necessary. Showers are even necessary when a person is in a good environment, because the mold that we sweat out of our pores is just as dangerous as mold that comes from a bad building or bad air. There have been dozens of times when a shower provides instant relief from symptoms. And outdoor mold toxins can be more powerful than you think; sometimes a shower is necessary even if you haven't gone in any buildings, if the outdoor air is bad.

And interestingly, I began to become MORE, not less, sensitive to various EMF's (electromagnetic fields). EMF sensitivity is said to be increased for some people when they detox mold, hopefully to come back down into a lower intensity later in the healing process. Even sleeping with the space heaters in the back of my truck began to produce noticeable EMF reaction; whereas before dumping, it did no such thing. We'll be talking a lot more about EMF sensitivity in this book. I later would discover that EMF's make mold and mold toxins much more intense. And that EMF interacts strangely with parasites and worms. In fact, there seemed to be a trifecta of interconnectedness between EMF, mold, and parasites.

In parallel to these observations, many long standing symptoms began to go away, including my chemical sensitivities – they just vanished. They didn't stay gone forever, but they began to wax and wane whereas previously, they had been constant. Eventually, they did go away completely.

For a small period of time, I began to crave junk food and simple carbohydrates, and eating as much of them as I wanted did not produce any negative reaction, which is unbelievable and also a fairly common experience among mold avoiders. I believe the body was craving simple energy for the detox process.

Our four week stay in Dragoon was just what the doctor ordered, but was cut short when the weather changed. Apparently, after unmasking from mold, many people become very sensitive to ambient pressure changes before storms. Of course, it is a known fact that approaching storms causes people to ache and experience symptoms. The mold avoider conceptual framework for why this occurs is that mold spores in the environment release their mycotoxins when pressure drops, and so this increases ambient levels of mycotoxins, thus affecting people with all kinds of chronic illnesses. This explanation definitely seemed to fit, because when a large storm approached Dragoon, all of the sewers on the property which hadn't bothered me before, all of sudden became noticeable and somewhat intolerable. Erik and other mold avoiders often use weather changes to vett out places and determine how much mold is in the surrounding environment. Similarly, any contaminated items someone possesses also tend to "act up" and become more noticeable when the pressure drops. After doing mold avoidance for a prolonged period of time, I began to notice that pressure drops are in fact a certain cause of mold spores releasing their mycotoxins, and that this isn't just a theory. It is absolutely the truth. Just another instance of Erik and Lisa seeing things that others haven't discovered yet.

Nowhere is perfect. Dragoon was great for us while it lasted, and helped us heal in big ways.

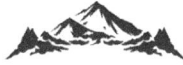

Chapter 15

TWO WEEKS OF ADVENTURES IN NEW MEXICO, ARIZONA AND UTAH

When we left Dragoon, we were rested, peaceful, had learned a great deal and experienced profound detox.

We headed east and ended up in Rockhound State Park in Deming, New Mexico. We ended up there after bailing out of a different RV park in Deming that crushed me with symptoms from a nearby powerplant; EMF symptoms which I probably wouldn't have noticed prior to being "unmasked" to EMF exposure. Thankfully, my EMF issues eventually calmed down and nearly vanished, an observation common among mold avoiders. Of course, people who never pursue adequate mold avoidance to kick-start the detox process may never experience a reduction in EMF sensitivity.

Rockhound State Park was beautiful, but we also noticed a new and different kind of biotoxin symptom here. This would be our first introduction to the symptoms of exposure to cyanobacteria, which is found in the crust of desert soil, as well as in certain other environments such as areas with standing water. Of course, Lisa and Erik do a good job of covering cyanobacteria in their books, so you can read more about it there. It is an important factor for mold avoiders. So back to Silver City we went, this being my third time there on this road trip.

This time in Silver City, my detox had decreased substantially and the magical, psychedelic glasses I had seen Silver City through last time (caused by circulating mycotoxins in my body) were no longer distorting my perception. This time, Silver City just seemed like a normal town. The dumping, metal detox, and healing continued in Silver City for 13 days, at a lower intensity.

We decided that we wanted to have some fun on this trip and show the kids the many beautiful attractions in the Southwest, so we spent a few weeks pursuing a fast-paced RV tour of the Petrified Forest & Painted Desert, Grand Canyon, Red Rocks, and a few other sights to see. We had some learning experiences along the way but mostly just had fun. We learned that dry camping, away from "civilidevastation" and away from RV hookups and sewer, was the absolute best thing we could do for our healing, despite it being the hardest way to live in an RV. We dry camped at Mather Campground in the Grand Canyon and also at Cosmic Campground in New Mexico.

The idea that staying away from civilization is the best way to do mold avoidance is one of the core principals that I intend to follow once our trip has concluded. I would love to buy 20 acres in a relatively secluded location, ideally above 4,000 feet in elevation and surrounded by pines, where my family can live and spread out and perhaps even try our hand at some small-scale farming of organically grown animals and vegetables. Ideally, we will be close enough to town to participate in activities and see friends, but just far enough to be away from the mold toxicity that typically accompanies civilization.

Of course, not everyone can live on acreage in the country. When people can't live in such a way, and are forced to work or spend time in bad areas, some mold avoiders have done well to instead simply attempt to spend as much time as possible in good locations. Some mold avoiders choose to vacation to good areas, or even choose to sleep in an RV in a good area between their work hours. Erik and others have purchased all-metal, small cargo trailers and do some minor conversions on them to make them livable, and then sleep in them out in the woods or in the desert, avoiding coming into town unless they need to. The metal construction of these trailers lessens the likelihood that mold will grow in them. Of course, the more the body heals and the higher one gets on the "power curve," the more time one can spend in bad areas without unacceptable health setbacks. In the beginning of the healing process, though, people often need to make more of a concerted effort to spend long periods of time (often months) being clear of mold toxins.

When further along in healing and high enough on the power curve, Erik and other mold avoiders have found that if they sleep in a really good area, such as out in the woods, and if they spend an hour or two a day hiking or outdoors in a really good area, then it allows the body to detox enough to stay ahead of the constant bombardment of mold toxins and other toxins encountered in civilization. This strategy would essentially allow someone to live a fairly normal life by giving them the strength to work, live, and socialize in society, while sleeping and exercising out in nature. It is necessary, upon returning to your pristine sleeping environment, to take a shower and "decontaminate," as well as change clothes, to remove any contamination that was picked up in civilization. Some people have found success without needing a trailer out in nature, and have been able to find good houses or apartments to sleep in. But it is more challenging to do so because of the problems that most modern buildings have and their tendency to grow mold. The best strategy for each individual will vary depending on how sick they are and what their life and work circumstances are.

After many people read this, they will be asking the same question. How on Earth is that a good life? Sleeping out in the woods in a metal cargo trailer? How can you say that is success? I asked the same questions of people who live like this when I first discovered this lifestyle. I got the same answer, over and over. Most of the people who are motivated to live like this are people who basically had death sentences before they discovered mold avoidance. People with such severe chronic fatigue syndrome, Lyme, and related illness, that they had to crawl to the bathroom. People with such severe dementia and psychological symptoms that they were being diagnosed with Alzheimer's disease and committed to institutions. People with such severe gut dysfunction that they could not eat or keep food down. For these people, mold avoidance is difficult, but it is a new lease on life. In fact, it has led to a much healthier lifestyle for many people who have left toxic cities behind in search of the balance and healing energy that nature offers. People often find themselves happier leaving toxic modern life behind in pursuit of a more balanced, primitive way of life. After all, all those "happy" people in cities may be a lot sicker than they look. Another massive benefit of mold avoidance is that it puts the power of healing back in the hands of the individual. Instead of blank stares from health care practitioners who can't help, we get to enjoy healing our own bodies independently. This benefit is so profound that I am still grateful for it each and every day.

This lifestyle also tends to inspire a new balance in other aspects of life, as well. I just can't imagine going back to the toxic, fast-paced, stressed lifestyle I had before.

As for me, the benefits and blessings of mold avoidance have far outweighed the inconvenience and cost. Each individual will have to make this decision for themselves. Certainly, the extent to which someone is willing to pursue mold avoidance will be based on the severity of their illness. The more disabled and close to death a person is, the more mold avoidance will seem like a blessing. To me, though mold avoidance has been difficult, it is so much better than many of the other treatments I've used, which submit a person to doctors, medical bills, toxic drugs, and many other repulsive aspects, only to still be sick. I'm naturally attracted to the simplicity and peace that nature offers, so the prospect of a new lifestyle of living in nature and camping and sleeping away from civilization doesn't sound so bad to me; in fact, it sounds really good. And as I said, many, many people are able to heal from mold illness without such extreme measures, depending on how sick they are. But when you are dying, like I was in that moldy home, each and every day of relative wellness is icing on the cake and the rest is just details. Feeling good again – body, mind, and spirit – brings me a level of joy that people with chronic illness just can't comprehend unless they, too, heal as I have healed.

Our fast-paced, 15 day adventure ended with a stay in Snow Canyon, where we learned even more.

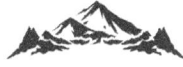

Chapter 16

SNOW CANYON, UTAH

Admittedly, by this point in our road trip, the lessons were beginning to wind down. We began to notice more and more that new experiences in mold avoidance were familiar, rather than intense new lessons. We welcomed this change. See, part of the purpose of a mold avoidance road trip is to reach the point where you know enough that further travels aren't needed, and you can bring the mold avoidance lessons and skills you've acquired back to your home town, or the place you choose to settle. You can then apply those lessons to living in your hometown; to finding safe housing, a safe place to sleep, and implementing good decontamination practices so you can heal and thrive in the community where you belong. For some people, endless travels may be possible and desirable, but for us, they are not. We have children who enjoyed our months on the road but who are now ready to rejoin their friends, their routines, their music lessons, and their regular lives.

Snow Canyon primarily taught us what it felt like to get "really clear," i.e., to be in a place that is so free of toxins that you can really experience what it is like to feel as good as mold avoidance can make you feel, at least at that point in time. We frolicked and had almost unlimited energy; hiked, ran, and played all hours of the day. It was a magical, blissful experience – and insanely beautiful, too. This was the way Earth was meant to be, and we longed for a full-time residence that could be located in such an amazing place.

We carefully took notes on what a super-clear location feels like, so that during our search for real estate, we could carefully look for these clues and make sure we didn't buy the wrong property. I presently have a long list on my iPhone of sensations and clues that are indicative of a good location. I consider my experiences, and these notes, to be a huge asset to me, worth more than gold. See, if I had known these things a decade ago, I could have been spared this whole ordeal. The whole idea behind mold avoidance is that we use our perception, and our being "unmasked," to carefully select locations where our body can heal.

We also learned that, as Lisa has said, "mold avoidance isn't always enough to get people well, and is often only a leverage point for other therapies to be used." We found this to be true as we noticed that many supportive therapies worked better than ever in this clear environment. All of the treatments that didn't work when living in mold, all of a sudden "kicked ass" during mold avoidance. I found that complex and tricky heavy metal chelation protocols were no longer needed. My body was in such high-gear detox that I could just take chelators randomly and have no side effects. It was astonishing.

It was also kind of funny. Because in our old home, we had access to tons of therapies. In the RV, though, we often didn't have access to much, but this was exactly the time when we needed our therapies! We laughed about this often. A good sense of humor was necessary during this journey.

Lastly, we learned that really good, pristine environments are not only places that *lack* toxins, but also places that contain the *presence* of a good microbiome. The modern, toxic world ends up killing off all of the healthy microorganisms and flora that are supposed to occupy nature. I strongly believe that a recovery from mold illness is greatly accelerated when a person is exposed to good, untouched, untainted biomes found in nature. The airborne microbial chemicals and byproducts from these natural biomes can positively impact and influence our own biomes, as we breathe the air. There have even been scientific studies on this, where it is discovered that people who live in different cities have different kinds of microbes populating their mouths, sinus cavities and intestinal tracts. If a particular city is full of toxic mold, what kind of organisms do you think will be growing in that city's inhabitants? You can think of places with healthy, untainted microbiomes as "probiotics in the air." A whole new concept, isn't it? A new paradigm. But it is, of course, much easier to stay in toxic civilization and take probiotic capsules, which is why no one ever talks about this, much less pursues it. Because it is hard. And it goes against our normal cultural trajectory.

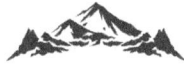

Chapter 17

LAS VEGAS, DEATH VALLEY, AND SURROUNDING AREAS

As our time came to an end at Snow Canyon, and we headed into Las Vegas (back toward Tahoe where we hoped to wrap up our road trip), the realities of our toxic planet began to sink in. I won't go into all of the details. We spent about two weeks traveling around and staying in various areas; Death Valley, Shoshone, Valley of Fire State Park, Pahrump, Amargosa Valley, and finally, Mount Charleston. Again, as usual, traveling in the RV gave us the unique and infinitely valuable perspective of being able to have CERTAINTY that changes in how we felt were not based on our indoor environment, but instead, on the outdoor environment. This is something that isn't possible when you are traveling and staying in hotels. The differences between locations were profound. If I told you about some of these differences, you wouldn't believe me. Our kids went from having bloody noses, bickering, laying in bed all day in some locations, to being happy, healthy kids playing outside all day in other locations. In some locations, I had a hard time walking down the street. In other locations, I was hiking mountains. Just imagine all of the sick people who don't realize that they would heal if they only moved a few dozen miles down the street.

The primary lesson for me in these couple weeks of travel is that everyone is different, and each individual must fine-tune the toxins that they must avoid to stay well or heal. Your toxins may be different than mine; based on our history of exposure, genetics, and epigenetics.

Specifically, I determined that there was some kind of extremely wicked toxin covering hundreds of miles in Southern Nevada and even parts of Southern California; a toxin which I believe was perhaps some kind of nuclear residue or even possibly a mold that eats the nuclear residue and produces radioactive mycotoxins. This toxin caused some pretty bad symptoms for me and rendered all of these locations fairly undesirable. Later, I would learn that a study found that Nevada is the most toxic state in the whole country, mainly because of gold and ore mines, and nuclear testing incidents. During my time in these locations, it was clear that my reactions were mold reactions. Not reactions to the poisons or chemicals themselves. And, this doesn't seem all that implausible, since mold is known to eat nuclear fuel. In fact, mold is known to use many strange chemicals as food sources.

It is interesting to note that many people who suffer from chronic disease and who have not yet been unmasked to the toxins that are keeping them ill, may spend years, decades, or their entire lives in regions with toxins that are harming them to an unthinkable degree, and never even realize it. Folks who who are badly affected by this Nevada mold toxin may be living in this region right now, as I write this, as their health continues to decline. They may have even traveled a bit and thought to themselves, "hmm, I think I feel better when I'm not in the Las Vegas area." But the shift is so subtle and seems so unrealistic, even fictional, that they write it off as their imagination gone wild, or as "something they had for breakfast" and don't do anything about it. Indeed, I admit, as do all mold avoiders, that these phenomena are often so subtle and hard to believe, that almost all of us wouldn't have figured this out if it weren't for the writings and help of those titans who have gone before us and paved the way, providing research and a road map. Because once you have the road map and can conduct informal experiments, it is easy to verify that the locations effect is for real.

Another confusing factor is that the changes and shifts that a person feels in moving locations can be so subtle, that they would be unrecognizable if a person were not traveling in an RV, converted cargo trailer, tent, or sleeping in their vehicle. Keeping the same sleeping accommodations from location to location allows you to sense differences in the outdoor environment, differences which would be drowned out by background noise if you were staying in hotels or Air B & B's. Moving around from one hotel to another introduces all the new variables of each hotel: is the hotel moldy? Is it a strain of mold that is worse than the last hotel you stayed in? Were the walls in the hotel recently painted? Is the person in the room next to you smoking? Did the last people who slept in your room sneak in a cat which you are allergic to? The list goes on.

By moving around in our RV, it allowed us to confirm that these strange and almost unbelievable shifts were in fact caused by the outdoor environment, and not something else. I believe that since most people in our country tend to travel and stay with family, or at hotels, or in some other accommodations, we never truly get to perceive changes in outdoor environments against the backdrop of an unchanging indoor environment. I would even go as far as to say that this single advantage was so critical in our learning process that the whole thing would have been a failure had we not done it this way. It is true that there were other challenges (many!) of traveling in an RV, not the least of which is the problem of toxic RV parks (due to their septic systems usually, as well as the chemicals people use in their black tanks, which can cause microorganisms in and around the RV parks to be particularly problematic). But even so, traveling in the RV became our "superhuman power" that allowed us to hone in on small changes in the outdoor environment, and to ultimately begin figuring out which toxins were the really bad ones that we needed to take special care to avoid. After all, one of the main premises of Lisa and Erik's approach is that it is impossible to avoid all toxins – they are everywhere. So instead, we need to learn to avoid the toxins which are most damaging to us personally.

This concept was a huge breakthrough for me, because obviously, the idea of avoiding all toxins perfectly is paralyzing, impossible, and leads people to inaction and being overwhelmed beyond all hope. But if we can get clear enough to begin to sense which toxins are the ones keeping us sick, and train ourselves to identify and react to those toxins, and subsequently avoid them, even if it means extreme measures must be taken (like moving away from hometowns and regions), then we can perhaps give our bodies the break they need to recover and heal. And the big surprise for me was discovering that avoiding these super bad toxins would actually cause us to become less reactive to the minor toxins and allow us to live much more normal lives. For example, after avoiding mold supertoxins, all of my chemical sensitivities went away, and many of my food allergies and intolerances went away. In fact, I believe that many people's food intolerances are nothing more than the collateral damage of living amidst mold supertoxins. Of course, it isn't necessarily a good idea to be exposed to a lot of chemicals and fragrances. It's not like I sought them out. But life became a lot easier and more enjoyable when perfume and diesel fumes no longer bothered me.

One interesting observation I pondered during our travels was the peculiar fact that people are certainly aware of SOME environmental exposures, but not others. For example, people filter their water before drinking it, if the water is bad. People try to eat organic foods. People often use organic cleaning products. People avoid food allergens. But almost NO ONE talks about air, and how the air affects our health. Why not? Do you not breathe all day long, even more often than you eat or drink? Of course, changing the air you breathe is much harder than changing the food you eat. So I do understand why this aspect of health is often overlooked. Nevertheless, such an omission in awareness may in fact be keeping you sick.

By the time we were done with our tour of this region, I was convinced that these two weeks had harmed my health more than any of the other toxins we encountered in our 4 months of travel. Yet, some other mold avoiders have felt that this region was healing to them. Hence, we are all different, and must drill down on which toxins are the ones we need to avoid. And though it is a strange concept, we need to think about the possibility that our whole illnesses, or at least the most limiting factor in our recoveries, is the toxins we are unknowingly being exposed to, either due to living in bad buildings or living in an environment with bad outdoor air or excessive EMF's.

Before moving on, I want to share a critical lesson I learned at one particular RV park during this time. We stayed at this RV park for only one night, but ended up not even making it through the night and leaving to sleep on BLM land at midnight. The RV park felt pretty good to me, and had almost no outdoor air problems. But it was located about 150 feet from a massive cell phone tower, and after a few hours in the park I began to have substantial EMF exposure symptoms. This was an important experience for me because, though I had had EMF symptoms in the past, they had never been so distinct and unmistakable. Again, being inside our same old RV – as opposed to being in a new hotel or new house rental – allowed me to be sure that it was something OUTSIDE, and not INSIDE, that had changed. By the middle of the night I was so wacked out that I had to wake up the family and we had to move.

The reason this was such an important experience had nothing to do with that particular day, or that particular region. After all, we would never want to come back to this place, let alone live here. What made this so important was that it added a new skill to my repertoire of avoidance skills: the skill of how to sense, and avoid, EMF's that are dangerous to me. This skill would mean that when we did find a city or region in which to settle, I would know how to pick a house or piece of land that was free from such EMF bombardment. It is also recommended that people purchase appropriate EMF-sensing meters, so that their own perceptions can be confirmed by accurate instruments. But this whole experience just underscores the broader purpose of the mold avoidance road trip – not just to heal the body and get clear, but to learn the skills necessary to pick a good place to settle down.

Of course, many mold avoiders experience a great reduction in EMF sensitivity, the more mold avoidance they do. Mold toxicity definitely seems like the controlling factor in EMF sensitivity. Mold itself is believed to communicate via electricity in some cases, and so EMF exposure may be irritating, or interacting with, the mold inside our bodies in some way. The more we reduce our mold toxicity, the less EMF tends to affect us. Of course, this DOES NOT mean that EMF is healthy for us – of course it is not. It may even cause cancer and contribute to the worsening of many chronic diseases. However, lessening EMF sensitivity is still a huge blessing to mold avoiders who are eventually able to live a much more normal life.

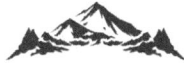

Chapter 18

BACK TO LAKE TAHOE: THE GOOD, THE BAD, AND THE UGLY

With a great sense of anticipation, excitement, and dread, we finally made our way back to Lake Tahoe. The plan this entire time had been to travel for 4 months and then return to Lake Tahoe where we wanted to live, and where we had lived for decades. In the back of my mind I knew that Lake Tahoe was believed to have particularly bad outdoor mold issues, specifically, the toxin which some people refer to as "MT" ("Mystery Toxin," as described in the book *The Beginner's Guide to Mold Avoidance*). Of course, the very worst thing that could happen would be for us to return to Tahoe to find that it was saturated with this bad outdoor air toxin. I can handle bad indoor issues: we could still live in Tahoe by staying in the RV and just not going inside bad buildings. But if all of the outdoor air in Tahoe was bad, that would be a huge problem.

And sadly, this is exactly what we encountered. Just as soon as we dropped into the Tahoe basin and reached the lowest elevation where the lake is, all of us began to sense one of the worst mold hits we had experienced in our thousands of miles of travel. It was a huge bummer and very sad. The emotions that we all felt over the coming weeks were extreme and intense and I won't write about them all here. But we were faced with not being able to go home, at least at that particular point in our healing.

This toxin is so prevalent in the Tahoe area that it is sometimes even referred to as the "Tahoe Toxin." It is believed that this toxin originated in Tahoe's history when a solvent spill somehow made its way into the sewer system in Lake Tahoe, and that other cities with the same toxin probably had similar solvent spills. Of course, this is just the working hypothesis about where this toxin comes from, and needs to be verified by science. This toxin is considered by the mold avoider community to be an outdoor supertoxin. The air seemed to be worst at the lowest elevations in the Tahoe basin, which sadly, encompassed most of the buildings and neighborhoods where we spend most of our time, including our church.

I spent several weeks moving my RV around to various friends' driveways, trying to sense where the toxin ended, so I could contemplate living somewhere in a higher neighborhood, or maybe on the outskirts of town somewhere. We even talked about how we could live up in a higher area and make minimal trips into town. I ended up camping in my RV on a friend's $7,000,000 property located on a private lake in a remote area of the basin. But I could still feel the toxin there, though it wasn't as bad. During this time, I also ran into what is well-described on the mold avoiders forum as a fire-retardant related mold toxin; that is, a toxin which results from the damage to the microbiome that occurs after fire retardants have been dropped onto forest fires. This toxin likely is emitted by altered microorganisms or mold that have been changed by the chemicals in the fire retardent formulas that are used. This toxin is also a very bad toxin for people with this illness. It is sometimes known as FRAT (Fire Retardant Associated Toxin).

It also ended up being true that the bad outdoor air toxin in Tahoe, known as "Mystery Toxin," has the capability of making indoor molds even worse than they would otherwise be. This phenomena has been well described by experienced mold avoiders, and it was our experience as well. So not only were we dealing with the bad outdoor air, but also buildings which were much worse than buildings we had encountered on our travels. This Mystery Toxin seems to kill off all of the normal, less toxic house molds, leaving room for only the most toxic molds to survive. A collusion of bad actors. A problem which compounds itself.

Some people suggested that we were crazy and we were just experiencing normal "snow mold" or "forest mold," but of course we had already considered this variable and noticed that other similar climates, with similar elevations and snowfall metrics, felt totally fine to us. What was going on in Tahoe had nothing to do with the fact that Tahoe was an alpine lake climate, and had everything to do with the problems in the Tahoe sewer system and with the use of fire retardant chemicals. The mold even smelled to me like sewer, though this wasn't something I was able to perceive before being unmasked. That smell and toxin easily contaminated my vehicle and some of our belongings, which is another problem Tahoe is famous among mold avoiders for: that is, that the toxin is very dangerous because it cross-contaminates items badly and is hard to remediate from them even after you leave the area.

The pieces of the puzzle finally started coming into focus as to why I had been sick for so long. As we drove by our old neighborhood where our mold house was, I remembered that there is a cell phone tower about 400 feet from our home. In our travels, we had discovered that cell phone towers – and most types of EMF – sometimes seem to make mold issues worse in near vicinity to the towers. While this observation varies among mold avoiders, it was usually our experience. One hypothesis put forth by a well-known physician to explain this phenomena is that the EMF threatens mold and makes it more aggressive, and causes it to produce more or worse toxins. While this is only a hypothesis, we did in fact find that our old neighborhood felt particularly bad to us. We all became ill and got bad headaches just driving through it in the car.

Of course, many of our neighbors were happy and apparently healthy and went about their business as usual. We stopped and visited with them.

This illness didn't appear to affect everyone. I don't categorically condemn Tahoe as a bad location for all people. These observations are specific to folks who have this illness.

It seemed to me that I was finally putting the pieces of the puzzle together. Yet, many of the factors which make locations and homes become toxic are unknown. Science is still very early in this area of study. This chapter contains my speculation about why our neighborhood felt so bad to us. But much research has yet to be done.

Our neighborhood seemed to me to have a trifecta of factors making us sick: the outdoor air MT and FRAT, the cell phone tower, and the resultant worse mold that was growing inside the house. Various scientific findings point to the possibility that even well-built homes without water damage can accumulate dangerous toxins if they are located in bad outdoor areas. And conversely, some mold avoiders have noticed that homes with poor construction and some water damage may not have much toxic mold at all in them if they are built in areas where the outdoor air is good. I personally believe that this kind of phenomena may apply to our own home.

Current building science and mold remediation knowledge would laugh at my assessment. Modern science and building wisdom doesn't recognize the authority of mold avoiders with heightened senses. And of course, I am not asking the world to believe me. I am simply sharing what I myself, and many other mold avoiders, have experienced.

While I was sleeping in my RV in my friends' driveways to test out different areas in Tahoe, clinging to a sliver of hope that we could somehow make Tahoe our home, my wife and kids were staying right in the middle of town in a home we used to frequent all the time. They all became progressively more and more ill. My wife had started getting a bad headache just as soon as we dropped back into the Tahoe basin, and her headache just lingered on and on the longer she was in town. She also began having brain fog and other symptoms. Mind you, my wife is normally a 100% healthy individual, with no Lyme disease or other health problems AT ALL. The fact that this

Tahoe mold was affecting her so profoundly was beyond incredible. The 4 month RV trip had unmasked even her. I kept telling myself, "Bryan, no wonder you have been so ill. Your perfectly healthy wife is even affected by this stuff. Imagine what your body has been going through with the added burden of Lyme disease!"

The kids also began having old symptoms again. Dark bags under their eyes, sinus issues, behavioral problems, and other issues. People suggested to us all kinds of alternative explanations, but we knew what was going on because we had been observing each other closely and in dozens of different environments on our trip. No other variables had changed in coming back to Tahoe, except our location.

I left Tahoe for several days and came back again. And I did that multiple times. To test the idea that Tahoe was really causing this. Because it was unbelievable. Each time I came back to Tahoe, I told myself, "that was all a bad dream. You'll feel fine back in Tahoe, that was not real." But each time, I didn't feel good in Tahoe, and I had the same symptoms come back.

It was a bitter-sweet time. The realization that we may have finally discovered why we had been sick, and why myself in particular had been debilitated, carried such a great deal of satisfaction and relief. After all, we had finally discovered a huge piece of the puzzle after years of failed attempts. But of course, there was bitterness in coming face to face with the reality that we probably couldn't live in Tahoe. This cut deep. Careers, relationships, church, community. I had lived in South Lake Tahoe for 35 of my 39 years. We were richly connected on every level. In a small town of 25,000 people, with almost 4 decades of residency, the prospect of "starting over" somewhere else was almost unbearable. I think had it not been for our faith in God, we would have really despaired.

We left Tahoe. We no longer live there. Currently, we are still looking for a place to settle. We are considering Reno, where the air is much better and which is still close enough to Tahoe that we can maintain some degree of connection to the people and places that matter to us.

Also, we have hope, and faith, in God, and in the future. We do believe it is possible that God might heal our bodies enough that we can return to living in Tahoe one day, or at least, spend more time there. But in the meantime, we have to preserve what matters more: our family, and a central part of our family is our health.

I do believe that if we had had less exposure to house mold, that the out-door air in Tahoe would have been much less of a problem for us. One hypothesis among mold avoiders is that exposure to bad house mold pokes holes in the blood brain barrier and allows the outdoor air to do more damage to the brain. Which can be avoided if exposure to house mold is kept below some particular threshold, which we obviously exceeded.

So what we thought was the end of a four-month RV mold avoidance road trip, really turned out to be just the beginning of a new season of life and a new direction that has yet to reveal to us an ending. We trust that God will prepare a way before us, and that He will lead us to a safe, fulfilling place for our family to live.

Looking back over my life now, I shouldn't be surprised that Tahoe was so inhospitable to us. Ever since I was a young man, I've always noticed that Tahoe felt "different" to me than other places. I was never able to put this together until after doing mold avoidance, but Tahoe just had a strange aura to it, that I used to just attribute to it being "my home." But clearly there was something else going on; something more sinister and definable than just a feeling.

I am often asked how we can deal with the trauma that has accompanied this series of events. All I can say is that it is better than the alternative. The slow progression of disease that I was experiencing – and which our whole family was experiencing – was not any way to live. Since being out of Tahoe, we've all been healing on many levels, most notably, physically. This healing is worth it. As long as our family can be together and heal together, it is worth it.

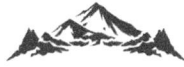

Chapter 19

A PLACE TO CALL HOME

I left South Lake Tahoe on my own, pulling our 33 foot trailer, leaving my wife and family with my parents while I went to seek out a better place for us to be. This was a very hard time. I literally took off not knowing where I would end up, exhausted and depressed. And, on top of it, I had to drive around with our huge trailer (actually, our home!) which made things even more cumbersome and intense.

There were so many criteria I had to meet in order to find a good place. Good air, no toxic sewer systems, low EMF, just to name a few. I knew that exploring brand new areas was super inefficient and draining. But there was no other choice at this point. I was also feeling a lot of joy at this time, because my health was better than it had been in years.

I didn't make it very far. After driving just an hour from Tahoe, I stopped at the Whole Foods in Reno, Nevada, for lunch. I felt good in Reno, and decided to make a go of finding us a temporary living situation here.

There were several attractions to the Reno area. The biggest of which is that Reno is very close to Tahoe, which would allow my wife and kids to easily remain connected to their support structure, community, friends, church, and family. In the face of living nomadically and so much instability, these benefits were huge.

Also, Reno offered a large variety of microclimates and microbiomes in a small area. The city of Reno itself is located at 4,500 feet elevation, but within ten minutes one could traverse roads to climb up to an elevation of over 10,000 feet. And, by making this short journey, one could trek through desert, alpine, and high alpine biomes. This elevation diversity not only allowed access to a lot of great hiking and mountain biking, which I had come to see not just as a hobby but as a satisfying and soul-feeding means of detox, but it also offered the chance to experiment with how I felt in different elevations and biomes. Plus, Reno itself is a relatively large city, with around 300,000 population, and offered a great deal of family resources, schools, churches, etc.

So, I parked my RV in front of a friend's house in Reno and began searching for a place to call home: a place to park our RV for a few weeks or months while we gave Reno a try.

Of course, again, I had some pretty strict criteria. After staying a night or two in the RV at each of the local RV parks, I quickly realized that they all were too problematic for us. High EMFs, moldy sewer systems, or cyano-infested water plagued them all. I had the idea to contact Air B and B's in the area to see if any of them would be willing to host a trailer on their properties, and I began to hone in on an area of Reno where I wanted to try living: Galena. Galena is a suburb of Reno located 1,000 feet higher in elevation than the city, right below the treeline of the Sierra Nevada Mountains. It was the perfect place: ten minutes from the city, but right near the neighboring alpine pine forest biome. It took me ten days of basically full-time work contacting dozens of Air B and B's before I finally arrived on a good option: a 3 acre parcel where we were invited to park our trailer in Galena. Of course, the property didn't have full RV hookups so I had to spend almost $1,000 in long-distance extension cords and a lightweight long distance hose, to connect to the water and power at the house. Also, I had to learn how to have our waste tanks pumped by a mobile waste removal company weekly.

The process of figuring this all out and contacting dozens of Air B and B's over those ten days completely wore me out and was pretty traumatic, since for most of that time I was completely unable to find a safe and healthy place to park the RV, and I was not with my family. I basically used every waking minute to make calls, and didn't even build any time into my schedule to grocery shop or cook. Instead, I pretty much only ate one meal a day; for this meal I went to Whole Foods and partook in their excellent food bar where I was able to eat a hearty meal and read ingredients for all the dishes. I very much hope that Reno works out for us longterm, because I NEVER want to have to do this kind of house-hunting again! (OK, well it wasn't house hunting, it was hunting for RV parking).

The positive aspect of this experience was that at least my wife and kids got to stay with my parents in Tahoe where they were pampered, well taken care of, and got to see all of their friends. So that made me feel a lot better about the whole situation.

The 3-acre property we were parking the RV on ended up being a great place from which to conduct our research to find out if Reno would work for us.

Being so close to Tahoe, we made several weekend trips up there to see friends and participate in our beloved "old" lives. Sadly, Tahoe has been extremely hard on me in terms of the damage done by the indoor mold as well as outdoor toxin known as "MT", or "Mystery Toxin." I believe that I am particularly susceptible to this toxin because of having grown up in Tahoe and my illness having taken root during exposure to this toxin.

We ended up spending 6 months in Reno, and learned a lot more lessons. After about a month back in Reno, we made the mistakes of buying new clothing at a known moldy store and Hell Toxin (HT) hotspot. People who have dealt with HT have noticed that it "explodes" (disperses all over a space) when it is washed indoors. In other words, you put new HT-saturated clothes in a washing machine inside your home, and it will scatter the HT spores and toxins all over the place. This led us to trade in the trailer yet again! So we were on our third trailer in just over 6 months!

We also rented an apartment in Reno temporarily and enrolled the kids in public school, but finally abandoned that plan as the kids began to show mold symptoms again in that school.

After we had lived for some time in Reno, I had sort of forgotten that it had been a really long time since I last spent time in a really pristine area. Mold avoiders have reported that spending time in a pristine area is extremely beneficial, but I had just started to subconsciously downplay this importance, as well as believe that I had "already spent enough time in pristine areas."

We joined up with friends on our beloved annual camping trip to what turned out to be a very pristine area up in the Sierra Nevada Mountains. This was actually the ONLY time I had spent time in a pristine area in several months, probably since Snow Canyon, Utah. It turned out that my body must have REALLY needed this pristine break from Reno life, because I started dumping toxins quickly and feeling much, much better, including renewed energy and some very large and respectable bike rides. Pristine areas tend to be a bit mysterious, but they usually have very clean air; are very far from civilization; are often high elevation; and can stimulate the body into spontaneous detoxification and sometimes even spontaneous remissions from disease. And ironically, this campground was the exact same place where I had experienced such great health boosts when tent camping at various times in the past, before I had even discovered my mold issues.

When we returned to Reno after 5 days of camping, I felt much worse. I am not sure, but what seemed to be happening was that my body was so shocked by the return to civilization that my detox pathways closed up promptly, and all of the metals and toxins that were released during the camping trip became trapped in circulation and in my tissues. This was my first run-in with what people call "mast cell activation syndrome" (MCAS).

It was frightening and horrible, and I attribute it mostly to the effects of unbound heavy metals circulating in my system.

On a leap of faith, I packed up our camping gear again and took off out of Reno, back to the campground, with supplies for a few days, and lots and lots of chelation agents.

I was desperate. That return to Reno from the campground had put me in a very bad place. I was hoping that advice I had heard on the Mold Avoiders group would save me; that is, that it is much easier to detox and clean the body of heavy metals when in a pristine location. In fact, some people reported that chelation agents which normally were intolerable and caused horrible metal redistribution, were actually easy to tolerate and very beneficial when in pristine air. Seems far fetched, right?

Well, this is exactly what happened to me. When I got back to the campground, my body started craving and energetically testing well for tons of chelation agents. I was literally gobbling huge doses of these agents which normally I could only tolerate in very small doses, if at all.

Substances like OSR, MicroSilica, Modifilan, Apple Pectin, DMPS, ALA, modified citrus pectin...these substances became my golden parachute out of a very messy and arduous metal stir-up which began when I went camping the first time and returned to civilization with too many metals still in circulation. Sure enough, my MCAS symptoms just magically vanished after this chelation pursuit.

My wife and kids met up with me and we camped a total of another 5 nights on this second trip. It was at this time that I realized that healing would require some focused, determined, dedicated time in pristine areas. And that Reno wasn't at all as pristine as I had hoped it would be, even way up high on a mountainside 1,000 feet in elevation above the city.

Back in Reno after camping, we continued to evaluate our options and try to make a plan. Winter was coming soon, and while my family was cozy in the apartment, I could only tolerate a few hours a day at the apartment. And since the trailer was contaminated with HT (this was before I traded it in for a second time), there was no safe indoor space for me. In fact, I'm writing this very chapter from the Burger King located inside the local Walmart, which, amazingly, feels OK to me. I spent most of the 100 degree Reno days without shelter, living outdoors, and sleeping in my truck. Thankfully, the new car we had just purchased for my wife – a Volkswagen Tiguan – was clean and felt good to me and I was able to pass many an afternoon just literally hanging out in the car with the A/C turned on. Many mold avoiders have also reported being confined to living in their cars for similar reasons. Much of this book was also written sitting on a rock, under the shade of a tree, squinting in the sun. So, forgive me if the book isn't as well-written as my other books!

As Fall neared, we had to figure something else out. We were paying double rent – at the apartment and the property where I was sleeping in my truck. And, as if this were some twisted comedy, even paying double rent (over $3,000/mo) and draining our finances, there was STILL no place for me to live indoors. Truth be told, the reality was that I couldn't afford to pay rent to two properties and not be able to live in any of them.

In fact, having no safe indoor space has a lot of not-so-obvious downsides. Besides the heat and discomfort, this kind of lifestyle is incredibly inefficient, and there's little time and energy for things like working, planning, paying bills, organizing life, and making future plans. Also having a great deal of fear about doing laundry inside the trailer and resorting to using a primitive portable washing machine outside the trailer, I found myself feeling a lot like an animal or a person living in a third world country. What would I eat today? Where or how would I shower? I went to Walmart several times a day and walked out with only a few items that would be provision for just the immediate needs. The human capacity of forethought, planning, and doing grocery shopping for multiple days, was just a level of functioning I wasn't capable of. Thankfully, the apartment gave my wife and kids a much higher degree of stability and normalcy. But still, we couldn't afford to keep paying two rents, and winter was coming. I had to figure out what we would do for the winter, and in order to stay in Reno, where temps can drop into the 20's and sometimes teens, living outside wasn't going to work.

I finally just gave up on Reno, at least for that period of time. We moved back into the RV and left for the winter. This turned out to be a really good decision, as we were able to travel in the Southwest for the second winter in a row, and enjoy good weather and proper RV living. I discovered that having a good RV and living in a warm climate in good air, is simply worthwhile, no matter what sacrifices are involved. Shelter and clean air can offer the peace of mind needed to work and plan and attend to life's challenges.

As I write this, we are currently in New Mexico in February, 2019, doing very well and scouting out possible places to settle.

Part III:

THE TREATMENTS THAT HELPED ME RECOVER FROM MOLD ILLNESS

Chapter 20

MOLD, BIOFILM AND BARTONELLA (AND WHY OZONE 10 PASS KILLS THEM ALL)

The previous section of this book was a travel diary which was written to share not only our mold avoidance adventures, but also the lessons we learned on the road.

The current section will move on to explore some of the various supportive treatments that I found to be most helpful during my recovery from mold illness. I will also be sharing some other lessons, observations, and tips I've learned, in no particular order. Please remember that these treatments were only helpful in the context of ongoing mold avoidance. Also, I will not be discussing most of the mold treatments which are already used in modern mold illness therapy, since these treatments are discussed at length in other information sources. For example, I did find that cholestyramine was helpful, but only when used in the context of mold avoidance.

Since I wrote my last book (titled *Freedom From Lyme Disease,* and probably my most significant book to date), the three most important discoveries I've made are: mold avoidance, ten pass ozone, and live bee venom therapy. We will take a look at those therapies now.

Let's start by looking at ten pass ozone. For a detailed explanation of what ten pass ozone is, read the blog article on my Anti-Lyme Journal website, at www.antilyme.com. The article is entitled, *New Lyme Treatment is Mainstay for Southern California LLMD*. This article also introduces you to Dr. Mary Ellen Shannon, MD, who practices medicine at the Center for New Medicine in Irvine, CA. She is the doctor from whom I've received all of my ten pass ozone treatments (I've had about 25 of them now), and I highly recommend her.

It is known that mold toxicity can make chronic infections of all sorts, much worse. A participant on the Mold Avoider forum proposed the hypothesis that the reason mold makes infections worse is that it acts as a biofilm to protect the infections. In other words, as mold molecules enter the human body, Lyme and co-infections grab onto that mold and integrate it into their biofilm structure, using mold as a building material to construct the biofilms.

The more I read and experienced after I heard this, the more I realized this was becoming my paradigm for understanding mold illness, and this explained why those with chronic infections seem to be most affected by mold illness. Sure, some folks without chronic infections end up with mold illness, but the more I watch, the more I see that a vast majority of mold sufferers also have such things as chronic Lyme disease, chronic viral infections, or chronic parasites. The connection between infections and mold became so ubiquitous that it was undeniable. Just about every new member of the mold avoiders group, sure enough, announced that they were suffering from chronic Lyme disease or some other chronic infections.

I am certainly not saying that mold doesn't cause other kinds of damage in the body. We know, of course, that mold is immunosuppressive, and that it also causes the blood to thicken, and causes hormonal disarray, and a number of other kinds of damage. It is a direct toxin in and of itself and certainly doesn't need to be combined with infections in order to do damage. And, the immunosuppressive effects of mold also open up the doors to infection. But for me personally, the biofilm hypothesis matched best with my own experiences. Each time I got a "mold hit," it felt like the infections were adding a layer of biofilm onto their colonies.

Another theme that began to emerge repeatedly in myself and others, was the correlation between mold and Bartonella; in particular, mold's ability to build Bartonella's strength and help Bartonella survive. This observation has been confirmed by several top doctors, one of whom released a leading 2018 mold book. This connection became more and more self-evident the longer I studied and dealt with this issue. Mold hits just seemed to add layers onto Bartonella colonies, increasing Bartonella symptoms and the necessity for treatment. This became a major underlying theme and direction for me to push in, over the months.

And this brings us to why I believe that ozone 10 pass therapy is so effective for combatting this illness. Ozone 10 pass appears to be one of the only therapies which addresses all three of these problems (mold, biofilm, and Bartonella) with swift effectiveness. This shouldn't be at all surprising, since ozone is a strong oxidizer and is known for its ability to just bulldoze through any and all impurities in the body. Other, less aggressive methods of ozone application can of course help as well, but 10 pass really was the only one that provided the kind of progress that really lead to healing, in my case. Before I used ozone ten pass, I was a very regular user of ozone rectal insufflation, ear insufflation, ozonated water, and even ozone injections into problem areas. But the ozone ten pass beats them all.

It turned out that the issue with Bartonella really wasn't that it was hard to kill. In fact, once the mold and biofilm were removed, Bartonella felt effort-less to kill. The hard part was removing the mold and biofilm, which almost NOTHING accomplished except ozone 10 pass. And as a bonus, many people have also noticed that ozone 10 pass also has direct killing power against Bartonella, and I would agree with this observation, though I think the more helpful part of the ten pass is the elimination of mold and biofilm. So, for anyone pursuing ten pass ozone, don't waste the opportunity that 10 pass affords you to kill the hell out of Bartonella. All those old Bartonella treatments you have that don't work anymore – they will all of a sudden work like never before. Even old rife frequencies like 832 Hz seemed to spring to life all of a sudden after 10 pass. So, bring all of your Bartonella treatments with you when you go get your ten pass!

Let me illustrate this by telling you my own experience. In Fall, 2017, when I was at my absolute sickest, I knew I was dealing with Bartonella, but no therapies had any effect at all in reducing the infection. Nothing: not anti-biotics, not herbs, not rife. But after my first few ozone ten pass treatments with Dr. Shannon, all of a sudden, all of those same treatments worked with swift and decisive effectiveness, almost instantly. It was is if my Bartonella was a weak, wimpy infection, and any staying power it had was all based on its ability to hide behind moldy biofilms. No wonder people still living in mold can't get better!

This also explains why common biofilm busting herbs seemed to do nothing for my Bartonella. Because most biofilm herbs don't take into account the mold, and in fact, very few, if any, herbs are even capable of removing mold from the body.

And while cholestyramine and other popular mold binders do remove mold from the body, I have not found them to be helpful in disassembling the biofilms that protect the infections.

Can mold avoidance alone accomplish what ozone accomplishes? The answer is a bit tricky, at least for me. I believe that yes, mold avoidance alone could accomplish the removal of the moldy biofilms, exposing the weakened Bartonella infection underneath. But the extreme and perfect level of mold avoidance that would need to be carried out in order to accomplish this is far beyond the ability of most normal people, and even most extreme mold avoiders, especially if they have kids. Uber-extreme mold avoidance may do the same thing, but it is almost impossible to accomplish, and ozone ten pass seems to "cover all sins" by allowing a "reset" button on mold in the body. Even if mold avoidance alone could accomplish it, it would most certainly take a lot longer. Like, hundreds of times longer. So I personally felt that ten pass ozone was a fantastic short cut. The ozone did not replace my need to do mold avoidance. It just helped me get better faster.

There was a time when I could feel my Bartonella and mold symptoms starting to creep back in, even after I had done several ten pass ozone treatments. This happened when we returned from our road trip and I was in Reno scouting out a location for my family to settle. At this time, it was almost impossible to prevent the worsening of mold and Bartonella, even with pretty darn good mold avoidance practices. Sure, I could have tried to be even more extreme and isolate myself from all societal participation and live alone on a mountain, never going into town. And, I certainly don't have anything negative to say about the mold avoiders I know who do it that way. But I came to a realization during this time: if a therapy such as ozone 10 pass is in fact available and could lessen the degree to which mold avoidance practices are required, why not use it?

As I pondered this idea (that ozone 10 pass could help decrease the degree of mold avoidance I would need to practice), I was reminded of my first ozone 10 pass experience in October of 2017. When I traveled to Oceanside to see Dr. Shannon that first time, I was in fact still living in mold and practicing zero mold avoidance. And still, just five 10 pass treatments had a profound effect in unmasking me and eliminating mold and biofilm. So this was further support for my hypothesis that ozone 10 pass could in fact do some heavy lifting, even if mold avoidance isn't perfectly addressed. The conclusion to the matter is probably something like this: the more ozone 10 pass I can do, the less I need mold avoidance. And conversely, the more mold avoidance I do, the less I need ozone 10 pass. So a person could conceivably mix and match the two therapies as they felt was most convenient and practical for their individual situation. But in the end, I became extremely grateful for ozone 10 pass and its ability to release me somewhat from the bondage of ultra-extreme mold avoidance. Less extreme mold avoidance is something I don't mind at all, and has actually led our family to a much more peaceful, balanced, and happy existence. All these observations have led me to believe that A LOT more Lyme sufferers have mold illness than we realize. Because, many Lyme sufferers can't seem to get better without ozone ten pass, and ozone ten pass is also just about the only thing that can remove mold from biofilms throughout the body. In fact, the more ozone ten pass I did (and I've done a lot of them), the more I realized that "Lyme disease and co-infections" aren't the primary problems in this chronic illness, but instead, mold is the primary problem. Lyme disease is just an opportunistic infection which happens to thrive in the presence of mold exposure. This doesn't make the damage caused by Lyme disease any less important. Lyme still causes damage and hurts the body. It is just that Lyme is only there in the first place because of mold exposure. It is a fascinating experience to watch the "Lyme layer" of illness be peeled away, as mold is removed.

I am not entirely certain whether the moldy biofilm protecting Bartonella is alive or dead mold. But I suspect that it is alive, and that one of the ways in which environmental mold exposures seem to do harm is by initiating some type of quorum sensing or communication, "waking up" the dormant mold inside of us. So by avoiding mold, we are preventing the mold inside of us from getting signals to be more active. This may also be why spending time in a "good location," also known as a "pristine area," helps us; because instead of mold communicating with our biome, we are getting communication from more beneficial, natural flora in the forest, and that causes the "good" organisms in us to grow and dominate the bioterrain. In this way, one can conceptualize the human body as merely an extension of the bioterrain in the external environment.

I believe that mold colonization becomes especially noticeable later in the mold avoidance process, after a person has done substantial detoxing. For example, after about 9 months of mold avoidance, I began to notice that bizarre mold-related symptoms I was having no longer were responding to detox modalities, but instead were responding to efforts directed at killing mold inside my body and avoiding the quorum sensing queues that mold hits initiated.

Of course, mold exposures also cause a number of other bad things to happen inside the body, not just the communication / activation of mold colonizations inside of us. Toxic mold exposure has dozens of negative effects on human health. And, it appears that Lyme and co-infections, and maybe especially worms, can use dead bits and parts of mold to create biofilm, as I mentioned above. So there are many things taking place when we get environmental mold exposures, and it can be a long and complex process to solve the puzzle. I certainly don't have all the answers.

In any case, ozone, and especially ozone ten pass, seems to be especially helpful in this illness. Ozone ten pass was the key that unlocked a lot of healing and understanding for me. Don't forget to check out my aforementioned blog post in which I describe what ozone ten pass is and how it is administered. You can find that blog post at: www.antilyme.com. I also have published a YouTube video in which I receive ozone ten pass live on camera, while interviewing Dr. Shannon. You can find this (and my other videos) on my YouTube channel at: www.youtube.com/lymediseasepublisher.

It appears that many people need to keep going back for ozone ten pass or they backslide. This has been the case with me, though the need has lessened with time. I believe that there is some phenomenon, perhaps an infection, inside our bodies, which makes us literally a magnet for mold. So, until this phenomenon is resolved, small amounts of mold exposure will reignite the circumstances in the body which called for the ozone in the first place. And so I have noticed that the more mold avoidance I do, the less I need ozone ten pass, and visa versa.

As a final tip, and on a separate topic, I have found the frequencies sold at http://www.dnafrequencies.com/ to be incredibly useful. I've purchased several sets of frequencies for various pathogens and every time, I am blown away by how well they work. I mainly use them on my EMEM-type rife machine. I've even found the mold frequencies to produce particularly beneficial results. You can purchase a book I wrote on treating Lyme disease with rife machines by visiting: www.lymeandrifebook.com.

Chapter 21

LIVE BEE VENOM THERAPY

Live bee venom therapy has been one of the most effective Lyme and co-infection therapies I've ever used. It is also available for less than $50/mo, and can be done at home. My wife has given me over 500 stings with live bees (not at the same time!), and I credit this therapy with a large portion of my recovery. There are several good Facebook groups devoted to this therapy; one group has more than 10,000 members. Some of these groups provide instructions for the therapy, which is beyond the scope of this book.

Eva Sapi, PhD, a well-known Lyme disease researcher at University of New Haven, Connecticut, conducted a study on the anti-Lyme effects of bee venom. She found that bee venom, and specifically melittin (one of the components in bee venom) is extremely effective in killing Lyme organisms. You can read the full text of the study here: https://www.ncbi.nlm.nih.gov/pmc/articles/PMC5745474/

It should be noted that bee venom therapy can be dangerous and cause allergic or anaphylactic reactions which may be fatal. I am certainly not a doctor, and I do not recommend that you pursue this treatment. Instead, if you wish to pursue it, I suggest you only do so under the care of a licensed physician, and that you follow an established and reliable treatment protocol, which includes having an epi-pen available at all times during close proximity to the bees.

I am not an expert in this therapy, and so I do not feel comfortable writing about it in great detail. I will simply say that it has been remarkably effective, and my regular readers know that I have used just about every treatment on the planet. I hope you decide to further investigate it!

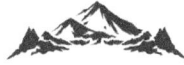

Chapter 22

THE CHALLENGES OF LONG-TERM HOUSING

I 've concluded that the biggest challenge with this illness is finding long-term housing. Modern building standards and code are often not compatible with the special housing needs of people who are mold-sensitive, and zoning and code laws often prevent people from living in alternative structures on their land (such as RV's, metal buildings, or specially constructed housing). This has lead many mold avoiders to have severe housing difficulties, even if they have the financial resources to afford to buy a normal modern home. In fact, if good housing could be found, healing from mold illness would drop on the difficulty scale from the most difficult endeavor I've ever undertaken, to simply a normal healing journey.

Some mold avoiders, such as a family we've become friends with who reside in Arizona, have become "fulltime RV'ers" and have lived in their 5th wheel for three years now. They can afford to live in normal housing and even attempted to complete a purchase of a new home, but ended up cancelling the transaction because they weren't confident the home would stay mold-free.

Many brand new homes have mold in them right at construction due to contractors exposing the unfinished home to rain during the construction process, or even drywall which comes from the factory loaded with toxic mold (yes, this has been verified to occur via independent studies).

Even if a house is mold-free at the time of purchase, it can eventually become moldy, which can then turn your life upside down again – both emotionally, practically, and financially.

I personally believe that people with biotoxin illness have a very good assortment of resources which can be used to heal from this disease (including Lisa and Erik's materials), with the exception of housing resources. In other words, housing still remains the missing link in healing and stability. This will hopefully not be the case forever, as perhaps lawsuits might be won in granting people the right to live in alternative housing on their own property, or perhaps builders will eventually start making structures that feel tolerable to people with environmental sensitivities. Until the problem is solved, though, I would be interested in collaborating with people who have ideas about this topic. I can be reached via www.lymebook.com/ct-bm-pg.

Before you email me, please realize that I'm not interested in talking about complex and detailed plans or instructions for building alternative structures, *unless* you've personally built and live in such a structure and it has been successful for you for at least a couple years. Because, one thing I've learned from other mold avoiders, is that alternative construction experiments often end up worse than conventional homes after a few years because these alternative materials are often unproven and while the plans make sense on paper, there is some unexpected problem that allows mold to develop later on.

I feel like the act of buying a home when you have this illness is similar to walking into a casino and betting it all. It's just too high risk for me, and so I really don't plan to own any real estate until my reactivity comes down to a level where I can tolerate more housing options. Or, if I do purchase real estate, I would like to have at least several acres to spread out and have the option to install various alternative structures without bothering the neighbors.

Also, I want to emphasize that I'm not interested in the "green tiny house movement" or similar movements. I do agree that environmentally-friendly tiny homes are a wonderful invention and I fully support the tiny home movement both in terms of its friendliness to the environment as well as its ability to set people free financially by reducing the cost of housing. I firmly believe that Americans have become accustomed to homes which are much too large and too toxic for our own good, often enslaving people into huge mortgages. But the problem is that many mold avoiders have found that these green tiny homes are often completely made out of wood and have the same susceptibility to mold growth as any normal home. This doesn't mean I am against the movement, just that it doesn't particularly meet the needs of mold avoiders.

Lastly, I want to point out that the housing challenges I have faced have been worth it in every way. Losing stable housing for a period of time, and even having to deal with primitive issues that humanity solved long ago (such as dry camping and not having access to showers and running water), has been a small price to pay for seeing changes and forward movement in chronic conditions which haven't budged at all under the influence of other therapies. Much of this book was written from a tiny laptop on the couch of my travel trailer, with poor internet and sometimes even inability to charge my computer due to dry camping and not having electricity. In my moldy home, I had a well-appointed home office complete with three computer monitors, a super-fast computer, and all the accessories that make work life effi-cient and productive. Yet, all that stuff became increasingly irrelevant as I felt like I was circling the drain due to mold illness. Working from a small laptop in a travel trailer became an immense blessing, as my health was turning around and I could imagine living long enough to raise my kids. I am telling you these things as words of encourage-ment for those who may be in similar situations, where pursuing mold avoidance leads to unstable housing.

Also, I feel that the availability of RV's and travel trailers is a huge saving grace in this illness. I can't imagine having done this without an RV. The

RV was the tool that allowed our family to stay together and pursue mold avoidance in a relatively secure and comfortable environment. We'll talk more about this in the next chapter.

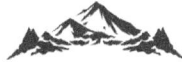

Chapter 23

LIVING IN A TRAVEL TRAILER OR RV: LESSONS, TIPS, AND LEARNING FROM MY MISTAKES

Because of the aforementioned housing difficulties, many people resort to living in a travel trailer or RV.

Personally, I have found my travel trailer(s) to be a huge blessing. They fill the gap between living in a tent, and living in a normal conventional house. I've slept every single night in my travel trailers and truck bed for more than a year. Not a single night in a hotel or regular house.

An additional benefit of this form of shelter is that travel trailers can be thought of as disposable housing. You can trade them in for a new one if needed, for a much lower price than trading in an actual house. Also, because of the small size of a travel trailer, they are much easier to take care of and monitor for problems, and generally easier to fix if water issues arise. And because they are mobile, in the early days of mold avoidance when you are a "beginner," it is much easier to experiment with different locations and not have the need to commit to a purchase or lease of conventional housing, which has the effect of locking you down to one location.

In fact, I believe the availability of travel trailers actually saved my life. It was an easy and effective escape route from conventional housing, and allowed my family to stay together and explore many fun and educational environments, while also learning mold avoidance.

When it comes to what to purchase, I strongly encourage people to consider buying a travel trailer or 5th wheel instead of a true RV. RV's have the motor built in, which makes them more expensive. Since travel trailers, 5th wheels, and RV's can easily "go bad" and become moldy, or become cross-contaminated with mold, or even wrecked in an accident, in my opinion, the most important consideration should be the cost of replacing the unit. The ones without an engine attached (travel trailers and 5th wheels) are much cheaper to purchase and replace, should the need arise. In fact, as I've stated, we did end up needing to replace our trailer (twice so far!) due to mold contamination, so I was very glad to lose only about $5,000 on each trade-in, rather than tens of thousands which would be the case with an RV. I should also note that each time we traded in our trailer, the problem was not active mold growth, but instead, cross contamination from allowing our RV to be exposed to bad mold toxins.

I also like to use a pickup truck to pull the travel trailer, and to place an aluminum camper shell on the pickup truck, which gives me one more option for a place to sleep should I need it. I utilized the bed of my truck many times for sleeping, during mold avoidance. For example, when our trailer had the horrible single night Chula Vista mold hit, and I sent my family to Texas to be with relatives while I figured things out, I slept in the back of my truck for about 6 weeks. The trailer itself was intolerable to me, so the back of my truck gave me a safe place to sleep while I sorted things out. (At this time I was still unable to tolerate most buildings, including hotels). We ended up trading in that trailer for a new one, which turned out to be a great long-term decision, but during the transition, the back of the truck was a lifesaver.

I also used the back of the truck to sleep in when we were in Dragoon, and I was heavily "dumping" and detoxing, because I wanted as clean of an environment as possible. The metal in the back of the truck makes for easy decontamination (you can literally just hose it down), and the very small space makes it easy to keep everything clean. I kept the truck parked next to the travel trailer where my family was, and spent the day inside the trailer and outdoors, and then just retreated to the truck bed when it was time to go to sleep. I was surprised to learn that most of the contamination which needed to be hosed down in the back of my truck came out of my own body! During mold detox, it is important to keep the sleeping area as clean as possible, and to decontaminate it often, since mold will literally be dumping out of your pores.

Also, the back of the truck has proven to be useful on many other occasions. It can be used to sleep in to test out different areas, to see if they would make a good place to permanently settle, since often, it isn't easy to feel out an area without sleeping there. It is a lot more covert than sleeping in a full-sized RV or travel trailer on a street corner somewhere. I've also slept in my truck when we are visiting family or friends, and their accommodations aren't mold-free enough for me.

In these ways, the pickup truck I own has incredible value to me. It serves, of course, as every day transportation. It is also needed to pull our travel trailer, and offers the kind of towing capacity to make our travels safe and trouble-free (I own a Dodge Ram with a Diesel engine). And lastly, it provides a safe and versatile place for me to sleep during numerous and diverse circumstances.

Some people are able to sleep in the cargo areas of regular cars or vans. This may work for certain mold avoiders, but it doesn't work for me. We are a family of 5 and the cabin area of our car and truck just get too dirty and take on too much contamination. Plus, you have to deal with all the new car smells, chemical offgassing, and VOC's. It is also much more difficult to decontaminate the cabin of a vehicle. I much prefer a truck where the bed of the truck is a completely separate space than the cab.

If you plan to sleep in the back of a truck, I have a few suggestions based on lessons I learned the hard way.

Use two layers of camping thermarest pads under your sleeping bag, as the metal bed of the truck is very COLD. I found these two layers to be more practical and comfortable than an air mattress. Using an air mattress in the back of a truck just sucks all the heat out of your body and makes it just about impossible to stay warm.

Also, use a cold-rated sleeping bag even when temperatures are not very cold. I found that it was always better to have too much warmth than not enough, since I could easily unzip my sleeping bag and open the windows on the camper shell if things got too warm.

When we were in Silver City, New Mexico, I was sleeping in the back of my truck when temperatures were getting down into the teens. I was parked at an RV park and used space heaters in the back of my truck, a few very small ones. This worked well, though you do have to consider EMF sensitivity; many mold avoiders go through a period of being very affected by electromagnetic radiation. Now that I've been doing mold avoidance for a longer period of time, most of my EMF sensitivity has dissipated or disappeared. With the exception of sensitivity to cell phone towers, and high voltage power lines, both of which I can still feel from several hundred feet away and which would be problematic for me to live near. But I have almost no problem at all with other forms of EMF, including the types of EMF we have in our trailer (TV, cell phones, laptop, etc).

I have compiled a more detailed list of trailer/rv tips, which I have placed on this website: http://lymebook.com/extreme-mold-avoidance. If you are considering purchasing an RV or travel trailer, I highly recommend you check out these free tips! I would encourage you to read and learn from my mistakes, and to spend plenty of time looking over this list. I almost decided to publish this list here in the book, but decided to leave it in website format so I can frequently update it, as I myself learn more about how to live and do mold avoidance in a travel trailer.

In conclusion, I have found that living in a travel trailer has been a tremendous asset to my family. The three trailers that I have owned have been perhaps the best investments I've ever made.

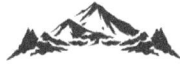

Chapter 24

MOLD AVOIDANCE ON THE ROAD VS. STAYING PUT

The idea of running around from place to place to try to avoid toxins has many disadvantages, of course. Living like this is extremely taxing, draining, and doesn't allow the stability and space needed to pursue deeper healing, work, and kids activities/friendships.

But moving around does allow someone to learn mold avoidance faster, and might even help someone identify whether or not their hometown is part of the problem keeping them sick. So, there are clearly advantages and disadvantages to moving around.

That is why it seems most desirable to me, at least, to do some of each. The traveling phase of mold avoidance really helped me to detox and learn about various climates and toxins in different regions. It allowed me to develop confidence that I could successfully navigate local toxins and find a safe place to settle down.

But when we do settle down, myself and many other mold avoiders think it is very important to continue to remain flexible and not get too attached to any one location or house, because outdoor air in any location is subject to change, and because any building or structure can always become a harbor for mold, over time. I know that this goes directly against cultural convention, where people tend to pick a house and stay in it for a long time.

So, for me, the best plan is to begin the process of mold avoidance with as much travel as you are able to accomplish, and then to settle down using your newly acquired mold avoidance skills. But even when you settle down, to basically be preparing for further moves that may become necessary. Maybe not moves to other cities, but at least moves to other housing. Personally, if we do end up purchasing acreage, I would like to have the option to live in alternative housing structures that are cheap, resellable, and swappable. Like RV's, or converted metal sheds. So that if a building on my property becomes moldy, I don't need to move off of my property but instead can simply swap out the structure. Pretty non-conventional, I know.

Part of the necessary preparation comes in the form of financial planning. Building an alternative, exotic, expensive mold-free mansion may be a very bad idea because if that home doesn't work out, it may have poor resale value due to it being so far from the norm. Mold avoiders should always build homes with an eye for resale value, in case they need to move. Renting a home or apartment would be even better from this perspective, if, of course, it is possible to find a rental home that is tolerable.

This is also why the compromise of owning an RV has worked out very well for us. RV's are by definition mobile, which would allow us to move easily. They are also relatively affordable and have good trade-in value, so that if the RV itself gets moldy, we can trade it in for a new one with minimal financial loss (especially compared to the financial loss of paying commissions to swap out of a home purchase). Living in an RV is probably not a long-term solution for most people, but for us, it has been a huge relief and a very workable short term solution for our family. It has allowed us to survive a very volatile and crazy season of life with minimal financial risk. And since we sold our home, and do not have a mortgage or lease to pay, we can essentially channel our housing budget straight into our RV expenses.

Of course, owning real estate, even if you don't live in that real estate, will likely continue to be a great long-term investment. We know more than a few mold avoiders who live in RV's but own rental homes, as funny as that may seem.

Lastly, Erik himself noticed that he never needed to travel very far to learn mold avoidance and escape the toxins in his city. Most of his learning and traveling took place within a 50 mile radius. However, this may not be possible if someone lives in a city or region where the outside air is bad over a larger distance.

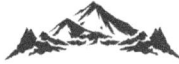

Chapter 25

DRAINING THE SWAMP: WORMS, PARASITES, AND THE MOLD CONNECTION

Many Lyme sufferers who have done lots of treatments and even many parasite cleanses come to the point where they believe their intestinal parasites and worms have already been handled. I had reached this point, too. But mold avoidance seems to really reveal and uncover many intestinal inhabitants who had previously been unreachable by even the most aggressive therapies. As you will see, this was my experience; parasites all of a sudden came to the forefront during mold avoidance. Also, it is now known that various species of worms, particularly the strongyloides variety, can actually disseminate throughout the body and live in the tissues of the body, not just the gut.

All of these worms seem to be able to utilize mold and heavy metal toxins in their biofilm and to coat their bodies, in order to protect them from herbs and drugs, and to help them evade the immune system. In my previous book, *Freedom From Lyme Disease,* I dedicated an entire chapter to the strange overlap between Lyme disease infections and parasite infections. I put the chapter online for you to read for free; simply do a Google search for "Lymebook parasites" and the free chapter will pop up. I strongly suggest reading that chapter before proceeding any further.

The more I participated in the Mold Avoiders Facebook group, the more a strange similarity kept arising among many members of the forum. No matter what their background or symptom set, many people seemed to share the commonality that they eventually discovered they were harboring an intestinal (or disseminated) worm infection. Some avoiders have reported that their mold reactivity decreased considerably when they eliminated the worms. After delving into this over many months, I decided I might as well give parasite treatment a try again, since I too may share that commonality even if I had already treated for parasites extensively and even if I felt I was already past this problem.

So, I began using some of the standard parasite drugs, which I describe in detail in the above-mentioned chapter. (For example: ivermectin, praziquantel, albendazole, diethylcarbamazine, etc). And in fact, I did discover that these drugs seemed to be a "whole different ballgame" after getting clear of mold. They seemed to pack a brand new punch. I also noticed that I began passing visible worm segments at this point in the journey, which had happened before but not as reliably as after beginning mold avoidance. I also began to notice that these anti-parasitic drugs started helping me immensely and making me feel much more like my old self.

Some anti-parasitic drugs are actually known to also have anti-fungal and anti-mold effects, which is a bonus. Living in the mold house, one side of my sinuses always became blocked easily and I frequently developed horrible, debilitating sinus infections. The longer I lived in that house, the more my right-sided sinus cavities became blocked and infected, until it was a daily way of life to simply never even disturb dusty items in the house for fear of getting a sinus infection flareup. Sinus infections controlled my entire life; everything I did was to prevent or treat sinus infections. NOTHING worked to cure them; not antibiotics, herbs, irrigation, sprays, nothing. My wife was ready to leave me because I would never let her clean or dust the house!

Mold avoidance amazingly cured my sinus infections. Gone. Just didn't happen anymore. But even mold avoidance didn't completely solve the issues in that right-sided sinus. I continued to have bloody noses on that right side, and some congestion and discomfort. Some new research shows that Alzheimer's disease starts in the sinus cavities, so this has always concerned me, since one of my main symptoms in mold was dementia.

A few weeks into taking various anti-parasitic drugs, I woke up in the middle of the night and I started having a strange feeling in that right-sided sinus. I got an irresistible urge to keep blowing my nose, over and over again. It was unlike anything I had ever experienced. It felt like my nose was giving birth to a baby. After blowing my nose constantly for twenty minutes, without knowing why, my nose proceeded to to release a massive, slimy object. It was the largest and most disturbing thing that has ever come out of my body. It looked like an infected mucus plug which had probably been in my nose for years. Apparently, other mold avoiders have had this experience, too.

I don't know exactly what the object was, but I know that even in the throes of the worst sinus infections, nothing as large or strange as this object had ever been released from my nose, despite taking those same drugs many times before.

But anyway, back on the topic of worms: The mainstay of my worm protocol is mold avoidance and anti-worm drugs, especially used during the full moon. Also, one fascinating protocol involves the integration of doxycycline into anti-worm efforts. Many established scientific studies show that some worms host a symbiotic bacteria called Wolbachia. This bacteria helps the worms stay resistant to drug treatment, and helps them process their food and reproduce. When you take doxycycline to kill the Wolbachia inside the worms, the worms lose their resilience and start to die, and become much more susceptible to drug therapy.

So as you can see, there is more to killing worms – whether disseminated or intestinal – than buying a two-week herbal parasite cleanse on amazon, and then thinking you are "done" with the problem. Most of my worm-killing efforts completely failed so long as I was still living in mold, no matter which treatments I was using to kill them. Which isn't surprising, given our knowledge that these worms tend to use toxicity to shield themselves from treatments and the immune system.

Another very useful tool: some mold avoiders treating their parasites have noticed that the addition of Mimosa Pudica, an herbal product, has dramatically increased the benefits of their anti-worm efforts. Some folks combine Mimosa Pudica with various anti-worm drugs to maximize results. It has been suggested that the Microbe Formulas brand of Mimosa Pudica is the most effective brand, perhaps because it is comprised of the seeds of the plant, which are believed to be the most powerful constituent.

The longer I did mold avoidance, the more I noticed that worms seemed to be an even deeper root cause of this illness than Lyme-related infections, though this is a tricky chicken-and-egg puzzle to sort out. And in fact, my initial illness did begin after an intestinal worm infection in the year 2001. That is what seemed to make the Lyme infections come out of the background and take over. It is known that these worms can alter the human immune system in such a way that not only allows the worms to survive, but also allows symbiotic co-infections to evade detection.

I conceptualize the relationship between worms and mold by using the phrase, "draining the swamp." We all remember Donald Trump's campaign slogan, "Drain the swamp." The imagery this creates in our minds is a deep, yucky swamp full of unsavory and yucky creatures. The creatures are protected by the murky swamp waters. By draining the swamp's dirty waters, we may not be directly targeting the dark creatures looming beneath the surface, but we will be exposing them, removing their protection, and weakening them. The assumption is then that they will be too weak and exposed to thrive, and they will probably wither away or leave. I'll leave politics for the talking heads, but I think this analogy works really well for mold.

I think mold accumulates inside our bodies and acts as a protective coating for yucky infections and parasites. Mold envelopes the infections and prevents other treatment from working, and shields the infections from the immune system.

By doing mold avoidance and pursuing active mold detox, we are "draining the swamp." We are revealing and weakening the creatures beneath the surface. This was not just theory; I experienced this exact phenomenon during mold avoidance. It seemed that actual mold toxins inside my body were shielding and protecting the infections and parasites.

I found one particular observation to be dramatic in this regard. Many mold avoiders notice that they become very EMF sensitive after they get out of mold. This was the case with me, as well. I wasn't bothered by EMF at all while living in mold, but sure enough, a few months out of mold, I began to be made ill by cell phone towers, power lines, and wi-fi signals (when multiple routers were nearby; the problem didn't occur with very low level exposure).

But I began to notice a bizarre, almost sci-fi like occurrence: That my reaction to EMF felt very much like a mold hit! How is this possible? I didn't have an answer.

And then, I began noticing something even more seemingly sci-fi: that when I took parasite drugs, the resultant herxheimer reaction *also* felt like a mold hit. So EMF, as well as parasite drugs, gave me mold hits; how could this be explained?

Over time, I began to realize that there was some linchpin, or some connection here, that was very important to this whole mysterious disease. Mold, parasites, and EMF: what ties them together? After months of observations and analysis, I came to the following conclusion.

My initial mold avoidance pursuit had drained enough mold from my body that the "creatures" (infections) in the swamp had lost most of their protection and coating, but they weren't going to go away quietly. They were desperately holding onto just enough mold "goo" to protect themselves, but they were living in a delicate balance, and the tide could shift in their favor or mine, depending on the amount of mold exposure I was accumulating. When living in the mold house, this battle was never perceptible because they were always winning and always had ample mold toxins such that I never was able to pull back the curtain and experience the draining of the swamp.

Let's start with EMF sensitivity. It is my belief that EMF sensitivity is experienced when the pathogens and possibly even living mold inside our bodies, are irritated or threatened by the ambient EMF, and so release their stored mold toxins into the tissues and bloodstream. Sometimes this may be an intentional survival mechanism they use, and other times it may just be the result of jostling and jolting them with EMF. And this is why EMF exposure gave me symptoms that were identical to mold exposure. Because the EMF actually *was* causing mold to be released inside my body.

And furthermore, when taking parasite drugs, I noticed the exact same thing: symptoms of a mold hit. And this makes sense, in the context of the current discussion: Mold avoidance had drained my swamp just enough that I was mostly feeling "clear" of mold toxins, so I could easily feel a dramatic increase in these toxins when the parasites were being irritated and killed by parasite drugs. When living in the mold house, parasite drugs were unable to reach deep within the swamp and so the parasites survived, and furthermore, if they did happen to reach deep enough to kill a parasite, I was so mold toxic already that I would have never perceived the slight uptick in circulating mold toxins... the swamp was already too full. But in a mostly drained swamp, it is much easier to see what the creatures are doing and sense small changes in their behavior. And so the final phases of healing involve wrestling with the beasts in the swamp who are now weakened but who are also retaining some level of mold toxicity within them.

Some prominent mold avoiders have suspected that parasites (and in particular, worms) are one of the root causes of mold illness, and now I had my own experiences to support this theory. Experiencing the mold-releasing effects that parasite drugs caused was a huge eye-opener for me and motivated me to continue extreme mold avoidance. Why? Because, obviously these parasites REALLY like and need this mold stuff in my body in order to thrive, and by depriving them of mold toxins (i.e., slowly "draining the swamp"), I was able to slowly turn the tide in my favor and start to win the war. Mold avoidance and detoxification allowed me to also utilize many therapies on the now-exposed creatures which didn't previously work. And it now became clear to me why *extreme* mold avoidance was so important: because even the slightest bit of mold re-exposure kept the swamp just full enough that this battle never played out and the parasites remained safely covered in their gooey goo, invincible against any efforts to notice or eradicate them.

Another fascinating observation I noticed is that Lyme disease itself, as well as the common co-infections (Babesia, Bartonella) seem to obscure the visibility of the above-described phenomenon as long as someone is still living in mold. In other words, a person may think they only have Lyme disease and that none of these other circumstances (mold, EMF, parasites) apply to them. This is how I too felt. Living in mold, I experienced none of this stuff, and had no EMF sensitivity at all. In mold, parasite drugs helped me a little bit, but not much. When I got out of mold and began extreme avoidance, deeper layers of the "onion" became apparent, for the first time ever. Lyme disease then became, more than anything, just a nuisance, something to be plowed through in order to deal with the underlying issues. Lyme disease stopped being the main thing, and started to be just a minor layer obscuring the deeper, more important layers. Do you see how important this is? So, if you aren't experiencing EMF issues and mold issues, as described above, you might consider the possibility that you are still surrounded by too much mold, and that you won't be able to observe and deal with the root issues until you get out of mold and drain the swamp. Even once I was out, it still took almost a year for the body to detox and heal enough that the underlying issues became noticeable.

A final caution: some people have found that killing parasites and worms can release a massive amount of heavy metal toxins into circulation. Lisa, in particular, felt that attacking her worms almost killed her, due to the resultant metals release. And so people should not pursue antiparasitic treatments without having a very thorough and comprehensive metal detox plan in place, and should probably save this pursuit until later in mold avoidance.

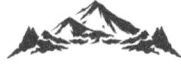

Chapter 26
ASSORTED OBSERVATIONS
ON MOLD AVOIDANCE

In this chapter, I will share a few other observations and tips I have for you regarding mold avoidance.

EXERCISE

Mold avoiders have noticed that exercise, and in particular hiking or biking up hills to gain elevation, has a valuable detoxification and symptom-lightening effect. This explains why I have spent the better part of my life seeking extreme hills to ride my bike up. When my friends wanted to do flat rides, I would very irrationally and angrily object. I always thought I was just strange for this desire, but I understand now the physiological root of it.

And so, exercise should be thought of as a very useful addition to a mold avoider's detox regimen.

MOLD MIND CONTROL

Mold can control you and make you want to stay in a moldy environment.

Erik has noticed that many biowarfare chemicals actually do their damage by convincing the victims that they aren't in much danger and should just relax about things. Mold is just like this.

I personally experienced this on various occasions when we used to go camping, and be away from our moldy home for a few weeks and out in nature, long before I ever discovered mold was an issue for us. I would start to feel better and notice changes in my body while camping. And within a few hours of being home, I would realize my house was making me sick. I would panic and take action, and talk to my wife about it and say "something has to be done." We even suspected EMF exposure at various times and spent a few days trying to live with most of our electronic devices and appliances turned off. A few times, I would even erect a tent in the backyard and sleep outside for a while after camping trips.

But somehow, almost as if a mad scientist was spraying our air with mind control potions, I would soon dismiss the possibility that the house was the problem. I would still be aware that my health was back to a steady decline being home from the camping trip. It was almost like I was telling myself, "yes, you are sick again in this house; yes, there is something wrong with this house…but it will be OK, just don't think about it or dwell on it and everything will work out." Totally irrational and nonsensical, right? And this happened to me at least half a dozen times. And I was never fully able to figure out what was going on. Some people have told me that in order to heal from mold illness, loved ones literally had to drag them out of their homes and change the locks. Seriously.

Of course, science has demonstrated many instances when parasites and microorganisms are able to control their hosts in order to increase their ability to survive. This kind of thing also happened to us even months into mold avoidance, when we would pull into a campground which we didn't realize was moldy. After a few days of getting sick there, we would some-how talk ourselves into the idea that it was all somehow OK, everything was going to be OK. This, despite intellectually *knowing* what was happening. The knowing didn't help.

This is an important caution, and should be understood and recognized! This single phenomenon, all by itself, may be keeping people sick, since mold seems to have the ability to turn off our ability to fight to leave and get healthy.

THE CHALLENGES OF MOLD AVOIDER LIFE

I want to address a very important topic with regard to mold avoidance. Being a mold avoider is the most difficult thing I've ever attempted in my life.

Being sick with Lyme disease was also incredibly difficult, but not as difficult as being an extreme mold avoider.

When I was first sick with Lyme disease, it was not a very recognized illness, and there wasn't much support for it. Many Lyme sufferers lost spouses and friends and ended up broke, and it was a hard situation to be in. Eventually, though, more and more people started recognizing Lyme disease, and there was at least some support and understanding among the public.

But mold avoidance takes the challenges to another level. You generally feel the same dearth of support that Lyme sufferers feel, but on top of that, you don't have the stability of consistent housing. I never realized just how central housing is to emotional and physical health. Without stable housing, it is just about impossible to undergo any kind of therapy for chronic disease. The anxiety and stress from not knowing where you will sleep on any given night is a whole different ballgame of difficulty from what I had ever experienced prior. Now, thankfully, I have gotten rather used to it. I don't even notice our surroundings anymore in campgrounds, and I laugh as our camping neighbors watch us do our laundry outside.

Indeed, the world is set up in such a way that conventional housing is really the only acceptable, affordable choice. Living in alternative housing such as a vehicle, tiny home, shed, or other alternative structure is illegal in most areas. Some mold avoiders, such as myself, who can't live in conventional housing, have at times felt demoralized, marginalized, discriminated against, and often hopeless. We are the only population of homeless people who are homeless despite being able to afford to rent or buy a home. And to top it all off, we are in desperate need of many therapies to support ourselves as our bodies go through rapid changes, healing, and detox from mold illness. It is very hard to focus on treatments when you might find yourself living illegally in a friend's backyard, or running out of time on a 14-day stay limit at your campground. It is quite a difficult situation to be in; the hardest I've ever experienced. And while we are sick and juggling these burdensome tasks, we are somehow also supposed to have the wherewithal of keeping our lives organized by selling homes, terminating leases, disposing of belongings, trading in moldy vehices, filling out address change forms, and tackling dozens of other administrative tasks which arise when moving. All the while from an RV, without a desk or even a printer, and often without power and heat!

The online mold avoider community becomes more than just a support group. The suffering and difficulty we've all experienced is so deep and fundamental, that these people become like family. They are literally the only ones who can relate, since most people with other kinds of chronic illness at least have stable housing, can go inside normal buildings, and don't lose their communities and churches.

Of course, I don't want to paint this as such a gloomy picture. I did all of the above with a smile on my face, because for the first time in decades, I actually had the energy and executive functioning skills to tackle it all effortlessly. But we still need to talk about it, and acknowledge that it can be a challenge. I think doing it with a family adds a whole different layer of challenges, as well. My wife reminds me of how sick I was in our home. And then I remember myself how sick I was. So sick that, at the time, moving out of our home into a travel trailer didn't even seem like a sacrifice. It was simply a last-ditch effort to not die. So, in the context of healing and recovery, unstable housing was definitely a worthwhile burden to take on. Yet, it remains the case that people with this illness are massively misunderstood and undersupported, and often lack the resources they need to survive. The government demands that homes and businesses can accommodate folks in wheelchairs, but no allowance is made at all for people with mold illness. And even worse, people who try living in alternative, mold-free structures on their own land, such as RV's and metal sheds, are breaking building code laws and are at risk of being told to cease and desist.

I very much hope that this changes, and that soon, society recognizes the alternative housing needs of this population of people. In many cases, the availability of alternative housing (such as an RV) isn't the problem; the problem is the laws which make living in alternative housing illegal. I hope and pray that one day, people with mold illness will be seen as having just another variety of legitimate disability, and that these people will be accommodated just as people in wheelchairs are accommodated. That is, that this population will be allowed to legally live in alternative housing while they heal from mold illness.

I am not sure about the correct way to advocate for this cause. There has been talk on the mold avoider forum about perhaps taking up this civil rights issue with the building and code enforcement government agencies. I would love for you to reach out to me if you have any resources or skills in this type of undertaking.

During our mold avoidance road trip, a friend of ours became paralyzed from a trampoline accident. Now, I'm not here to declare which ailment is more difficult to endure: paralysis or mold illness. I think they are too different to compare, and present very different challenges. However, I noticed that our friend received endless support from the community. Hundreds of people going out of their way to help. Tens of thousands of dollars raised in Go Fund Me campaigns. I'm very happy that our friend received this kind of support, of course.

But with mold illness, there's no support. Or at best, little support. At worst, condemnation, judgement, and shunning from family and friends. Homes are sold in emergencies at below market value, often with ugly mold disclosures. People are scrambling, living in tents and racing to buy RV's without fully researching them. Often, jobs are lost without unemployment benefits. I'm not complaining. I just think this is something we need to have open dialogue about.

BIG DECISIONS

If you end up being the kind of mold avoider who needs to take extreme measures to get away from mold (and I think more people fall into this category than the category of people who can just move across the street into a different house), then one of the best pieces of advice I have for you is to delay big decisions with regard to housing and even other life logistics. This is, of course, not originally my advice; I heard it from wise, experienced mold avoiders who went before me.

After getting out of mold (and you'll read about this in *The Beginner's Guide to Mold Avoidance*), you'll go through a period called "intensification," where your body will be healing and changing so quickly, and your reactivities will be varying so wildly, that it can be financial suicide to make big decisions like committing to long-term leases or buying a new home. Of course, selling the old moldy home you lived in is probably a good idea, still, if you are convinced you won't be able to move back in. Most of us shouldn't move back into that original home, so this is a safe "big decision", I think. But for some people, even delaying that decision may be wise.

It can be tempting to crave stability and just jump into the next thing, but if you are like most people and financial resources are limited, you may end up making a huge mistake. It is also not recommended to immediately give away or sell all of your belongings. It is a better course of action to put everything in storage and return to it at a later date, when you are more experienced at mold avoidance.

This is one reason why I really like the RVs. As I write this, I'm renting space on some remote land near Reno (in order to be away from RV park toxins). I'm living in my RV, while my family is living 10 minutes down the road in an apartment we rented. They are on a month-to-month lease, and so am I. We don't have any long-term housing commitments, and we can adjust our situation as needed. We don't own a home anymore, we don't have long-term leases, and we can just sort of hang out and wait until the right situation presents itself. Even moldy RV's can be handled with relative ease (compared to real houses) by trading them in.

Our lives are set up so that we can change things if we need to, quickly, with minimal financial loss. It takes quite a bit of self discipline to delay big decisions when you are desperate for stability after being ejected from your moldy home, but it is worth the endurance and sacrifice.

Also, I've been conceptualizing my safe place as a smaller and smaller area. Here's what I mean: If a person tries to maintain a completely uncontaminated and non-moldy, larger area, like an entire home, with kids and a family, it can become extremely stressful and risky. In our new connectivity with the mold avoider community, I've talked to MANY folks who have had to leave custom built mold-free homes because of a catastrophic cross contamination or other issues. Interestingly, these scenarios typically don't involve the expected water leak and active mold growth; rather, they involve a severe cross contamination of a mold toxin, most notably, Hell Toxin.

So then some of these folks are forced to sell their custom mold-resistant homes, and the market for these homes can be challenging, so more financial losses may be incurred at resale time. Not to mention the life stress of trying to keep small children pristine all the time when they are home, so as to avoid contaminating the whole house.

Rather, what I would like to envision being a better idea, is to think of the housing as a somewhat "lost cause." Hopefully it will be possible to rent or purchase housing that is tolerable to the sickest member of the family for visits and hanging out, but I would like to avoid enforcing strict and stressful rules about the house. Then, I would like to have a separate space, and to keep this separate space super clean. The smaller the separate space, the better, to reduce stress and upkeep. Perhaps a small shed, or mother-in-law unit, or travel trailer / RV, on the property, where I can go to "get clear", decontaminate, sleep, and work. Ideally, this separate space wouldn't even have too much plumbing or utilities like A/C or ducted heating, to avoid problems. Then, I would love to use an outdoor shower attached to the home, and if possible, use the toilets inside the home, to keep my space as simple as possible. Because I've been learning that it is just too difficult to keep an entire house pristine.

Of course, the main house must be good enough that I can spend time in it. But even in our RV, I often just sit on a metal folding chair while we watch a family movie, instead of sitting on the couch or dinette cushions. It's much easier for me to just have my own separate seat, than it is to worry about keeping everything completely decontaminated.

This also is smart financially because it would allow a person to purchase or rent a normal home, not a custom mold-resistant home, and that normal home would be expected to have normal resale value, and wouldn't involve the use of expensive and non-conventional materials that don't do well in resale value-recapture.

Of course, there are downsides to my approach. The main one is less family time, since there are inevitably two separate spaces. But I feel there are ways to mitigate this, such as having the family TV and games, etc, in my safe space, where the family will decontaminate and come out for family time.

Taking this concept to an even higher level, I'm hoping that my recovery progresses enough that my safe space can get smaller and smaller, until one day perhaps, I can consider hiking and sleeping to be the only safe spaces I need. This has, in fact, happened for multiple mold avoiders, so I do think it is possible. Though, it does require a good deal of getting "really clear" on the front end of mold avoidance so the body can heal enough, and stay high enough on the "power curve," to be capable of needing less safe time. I do think that sleeping is a key part of the day where a very clean environment will probably always be needed.

One tricky aspect of this plan which everyone should be aware of is EMF concerns. It is possible to manage mold cross contamination in a house and a trailer or shed in the backyard, but if a whole neighborhood is saturated in EMF, there's absolutely no way I've found to mitigate this to my satisfaction. I've tried a few EMF mitigating gadgets, and they don't help at all. And of course, we know that the new 5G cell towers are being rolled out. When I'm sleeping in my trailer on this remote land with very low EMF, I have learned to consider this an essential aspect of recovery. And this is why our current apartment situation isn't ideal and can't be a long-term plan; because the EMF at the apartment is so bad that I can't spend more than a few hours there without backsliding in my healing a great deal. And of course, apartments don't have trailer parking or room for a shed. But even if they did, it wouldn't help me. I STRONGLY caution people who are healing from mold illness from leasing an apartment. EMF sensitivity sometimes increases when doing mold avoidance and healing. In fact, I personally find that bad EMF hits at the apartment take me down almost more severely than bad mold hits, though I don't find EMF in other buildings or regions to be at all as bad, so I think it is a specific problem with apartment complexes due to the density of WiFi routers.

So, I think our apartment days will be short, and we will move to a more remote rental soon which may have some mold but which will be low in EMF. Or, hopefully, we will buy our own land soon.

But as you can see, there are A LOT of considerations when it comes to making big decisions, and it is best to let the learning curve run its course for a while (a couple years, perhaps) before thinking you can set down roots and make long term financial decisions. Of course, this is why I've always felt this illness would be so much easier if a person were wealthy. Since the housing aspects of this illness are so expensive, a wealthy person could much more easily deal with mistakes. But for most of us, chronic illness has already drained our bank accounts enough that we certainly aren't wealthy, and may not even have any degree of financial strength at all. It may be very hard to recover from housing mistakes.

BRAIN RETRAINING

At the time I wrote this book, probably the most popular, and most controversial, therapy available for mold illness is "brain retraining." I won't list the specific programs or companies that offer this service, but you can easily find them.

So, I want to address this topic. Basically, the idea behind brain retraining is that there was an initial toxic insult to the body -- likely, living in a moldy house. And, most of those who advocate for brain training do in fact agree that you should get away from this toxic insult. But, they state, after people get away from the moldy house, the limbic system in the brain just keeps on reacting, long after the toxins are no longer present in sufficient quantities to do damage. In other words, the reactions the brain has just won't turn off. So the brain needs to be "retrained" to calm down and not react anymore.

The question we are really asking here, is: Are the toxins someone is being exposed to just causing an over-reaction or allergy, like pine pollen does? Because we can safely treat a pine pollen allergy with antihistamines even if the person has ongoing exposure to pollen. We know that the pollen itself isn't dangerous. However, on the other hand, let's take someone who is being poisoned at work with dangerous industrial chemicals. Or someone who accidentally ingests arsenic or rat poison. This is a very different situation than the person with a pine pollen allergy, right? The treatment for this person is to remove the chemicals, or poison; not lesson the symptoms of the poison exposure and teach the brain to relax. Do you see the dichotomy? Imagine if someone was eating rat poison and their doctor told them to just retrain their brain to not react to rat poison.

I am pretty sure we can all agree that there IS a threshold of REAL toxicity that can harm us, for many toxic substances. Chemicals can euthanize animals in seconds. Even things like non-organic food, petrochemicals, and cigarette smoke are KNOWN to be objectively harmful to us. Is mold more like a pine pollen allergy, or more like the chemicals they use to euthanize animals? I realize my animal analogy here is a bit over-the-top, but I'm using it to bring some clarity to this debate.

I'll share my personal experience with brain retraining, and several hypotheses I've developed to explain these experiences. I don't want you to read more into it than that. I don't really think enough is known about brain retraining for ANYONE to make a conclusive proclamation about this topic. Instead, I think what we have right now is a lot of theory based on a lot of personal experiences. Of course, the science of neuroplasticity is well established, but what we don't yet know is how badly these toxins are hurting us, versus how much our bodies are simply over-reacting to them. But in any case, I don't claim to have all the answers, and each person is different. So understand that this is just my own interpretation of the available data, as well as my own experiences.

Personally, I have noticed that brain retraining is sometimes helpful, and sometimes counterproductive. The more I learn about mold illness and brain training, the more I'm convinced that there are actually TWO types of reactivity that are occurring with this illness. One type which brain training helps with, and another type which brain training hasn't seemed to work for.

Before going on, I want to make it clear that what I'm discussing here are mycotoxins specifically. Many people have also used brain retraining to heal from other kinds of illnesses and reactivities, such as MCS (Multiple Chemical Sensitivity). I believe that brain retraining might be useful in those other instances, but I feel that the science of what is taking place with mold reactivity in particular is a separate topic. I believe that mold toxins play a very special role in this illness, and to group mold toxins together with other types of toxins would be a huge mistake. One thing that Erik observed is that mold toxins seem to be the "master toxin," and that by avoiding mold and successfully detoxing mold, people notice that their other reactivities and sensitivities start to go away. The reactivities which diminish and go away include food sensitivities, chemical sensitivities, and things like allergies. It has absolutely been my experience that this is precisely what happens. Myself, and many other mold avoiders, have noticed that their chemical sensitivities miraculously diminish or in some cases disappear, when mold is removed from the picture.

On the other hand, endless pursuit of avoiding foods, avoiding chemicals, and avoiding allergens did me no good at all. Avoiding all of these things did not help me to heal and did not result in any decreased reactivity to mold. So you can see here that mold toxins are special. I don't think they should be discussed in the same way that these other toxins are discussed.

So, back to the two types of reactivity to mold toxins. The most damaging type of mold reactivity, and the one which brain training hasn't helped me with, is related to the chronic infections that most mold illness patients are known to have. Simply stated, I feel like mold exposures are somehow actually directly helping the infections in my body to regroup, survive, and remain inside my body despite treatment. There seem to be a number of ways in which mold is able to do this, including immune suppression and possibly even providing raw building blocks for the infections to use in creating its biofilm. I have also heard several other sources propose the possibility that infections, especially Bartonella, can use mold molecules to build biofilm. And so this type of interaction between mold and the infections seems to be more or less independent from anything the brain can do to help the situation. Also, many types of mycotoxins have been studied and are capable of inflicting direct, severe damage to human cells and tissues, even without infections present. So, these kinds of mold reactivity are the first type I am going to talk about. This is the "rat poison," not the "pollen allergy."

On the other hand, the second type of mold reactivity does seem to be related to a hypersensitive limbic system that isn't just reacting to toxins, but may also be "freezing up" and shutting down detox inside the body. I have noticed that when I do brain retraining, sometimes I can feel the body release mycotoxins which the body seemed to be holding onto. And so I do think that brain retraining has been helpful for this type of reactivity. But even so, it hasn't seemed to help at all with the first type of reactivity. And also, brain retraining only seems to be helpful, at least to me, for quite small amounts of mold. The larger quantities of mold seem to quickly overwhelm the ability for brain retraining to intervene. Remember that the body *intentionally* shuts down detox when too much mold is present in the environment. If I am actually being faced with too much mold exposure, and I try to do brain retraining, then I actually notice that brain retraining seems to harm me. It seems to attempt to outsmart the body and force the body to allow mycotoxins to come in and do their damage.

In other words, brain retraining seems like a manual override switch. It defeats the body's wisdom and lets mold in, when the body is trying to keep mold out. On a few instances, employing brain retraining led me to have very serious relapses. These weren't healing reactions or detox reactions. These were instances when I outsmarted my body and the mold that was let in damaged me, in the same way that rat poison damages rats.

I think one of the reasons that there is so much passionate disagreement about this topic is that people are all falling onto different parts of the continuum in terms of how much their reactivity is due to infections and actual damage from mycotoxins, versus how much of it is due to an over-active limbic system. There are some mold illness patients who swear by the program and say that it gave them their lives back, and others who have consistently pointed to the fact that brain retraining caused them to ignore exposures and have serious relapses. Both groups of people have, according to my observation, diligently followed the programs, and I think it is unfair to claim that one or the other group "must have done it wrong," because that hasn't been my observation at all.

We just aren't seeing much middle ground. People are either really helped by the brain training programs, or they seem to be really injured by them. I could be wrong, but this leads me to believe that this is much more of a nuanced situation than we realize.

Here's the thing: I believe both of the groups of people, with their opposite claims! I think it is a huge mistake to turn this debate into a polarized dichotomy. Many of the people I talk to try to push one of two absolute agendas. One group says brain retraining is the absolute answer and can work for everyone, all the time. The other group generally dismisses brain retraining as being unable to help at all. Just like with any other health topic, I think that black-and-white answers are rarely accurate. People and their situations, and infections, are very different. There are A LOT of variables that are different from person to person, including, how long someone has been sick and exposed to mold, what kind of mold they were exposed to, which infections they are dealing with, their underlying personality and emotional stress and tendencies, their nutrition, genetics, and other factors. So I really think the problem with the debate is the absolutism that is often displayed among people discussing this.

I'll continue to share my experience. It is incredibly clear to me that these toxins, in and of themselves, regardless of what the brain does, are highly toxic and can activate and incite infections, cause immunosuppression, and do direct damage to the body. Here's one example:

One of Erik's principles is that the body won't detox unless it is in a good environment. Which includes taking "detox showers" after getting mold hits, so that the skin is clear of mycotoxins. For me, I can feel my detox processes turn on almost instantly after a shower, assuming there was a mold exposure that day.

But I've also experimented with brain retraining at times when I know I've had a bad mold exposure, and when I know my body is covered in mycotoxins. I've actually been successful, during these times, in calming my body down and allowing detox to turn back on, while I'm still contaminated. Turning detox back on inside the body is one of the primary goals of brain training. I've done this experiment many times; dozens of times. And without fail, what happens every single time, is that my body does in fact turn the detox process back on, but at the same time, those mycotoxins on my skin immediately start to make me very sick and cause infection flare ups, sometimes, even severe flare-ups.

It almost feels as though the increased detox activity opens the gate for those mycotoxins to be absorbed through the skin. After this happens, I get quite sick, and not in a "detox/healing" sort of way.

So it does in fact appear to be a two-way street: that when the body opens up detox channels for mycotoxins to exit, these channels also allow mycotoxins to *enter*, as well (to enter sensitive tissues, cells, and the brain). And this is exactly what Erik has said all along – that it is a two-way street.

So there is a REASON the body has turned off detox processes when being exposed to mold. The body knows that letting toxins out means also letting toxins in, and the body isn't willing to make that trade-off. And so I don't think my limbic system is overreacting at all.

But after I do shower, I can do brain retraining just fine. And I do feel that it can turn on the detox processes in the body, in fact.

And so I do feel that the black-and-white, yes-or-no debates that are taking place around brain retraining are really counter-productive and non-scientific. Because I think there are a lot of nuances in what is taking place here, and the passion and fervency is missing the sane middle ground. So, as you can see, I think the false dichotomy in much of the debate is counterproductive. It kind of reminds me of watching political debates. Can't we be reasonable and understand the middle ground?

As for me, the city I'm from is believed to have some of the most harmful mold toxins, according to reports from many mold avoiders. And I was also extremely sick when we left the city. So, at least for me, brain training in this city proved to be more harm than help. These toxins aren't just found indoors, but also outdoors. I found that exposure to this "bad stuff" continued to mess me up badly no matter what I did with my brain. There have never been formal studies to determine if, perhaps, the people who benefit most from brain retraining maybe live in better, less toxic cities? This is a question I have often pondered.

On the other hand, I had a different experience wherein I was mountain biking and encountered some trees and foliage that was similar to the vegetation in my hometown where I became sick. My body immediately freaked out and went into fight-or-flight mode. Inflammation was activated in my system. I instantly recognized this as a perfect opportunity to employ brain retraining. As the ideology teaches, I dug deep into happy memories of when I had smelled and felt those same plants, and had normal and happy life experiences when surrounded by them. And, almost instantly, the symptoms lifted, and I felt a sense of calm and strength, and since that day, those plants and trees have never bothered me again. Of course, people *shouldn't* be reacting to plants and trees, so that seemed to be the perfect opportunity to employ brain training. Again, the brain retraining debate is nuanced. It isn't black and white. Which kinds of toxins are we dealing with? Pine pollen or rat poison?

Some brain training advocates have stated that "sick people" should be able to handle the same exposures as "healthy people," and if they can't, then the brain is over-reacting. However, I do not believe this is a realistic expectation of sick people. Every one of us has different genetics and biological stressors, and are susceptible to different disease processes. Some people can smoke cigarettes until they are age 100, and not get cancer. Other people get lung cancer after a few years of smoking. Should we expect that everyone should be able to smoke and not get cancer? Is getting cancer a malfunction within the brain that we can train away with brain exercises? Is one person's ability to stay healthy under certain stressors indicative that other people can handle the same stressors? Here's another observation: those who are in the process of getting cancer from smoking may have in fact trained their brains to not react to cigarette smoke in a negative way. Does this keep them safe from cancer? This is, of course, ridiculous. But asking these questions can help us become more reasonable with this debate. After all, mycotoxins *are* proven to be damaging in *real* ways, just like smoking is. So why are we pretending that people shouldn't be damaged by mycotoxins? It is somewhat insane, if you ask me.

So, again, my answer when people ask what I think of brain retraining is… "it is nuanced, and different for everyone, depending on a lot of factors."

Brain retraining, in my opinion, actually is very valuable and promising! I just get frustrated when it is discussed without paying respect to the nuances and details of the situation. I think there are better answers when someone fails to benefit from brain retraining, instead of the answer often given by brain retraining advocates: "they just weren't doing it right." This is such a cop-out and unthoughtful response. I also speak with many mold sensitive people who tried brain retraining and yet kept experiencing a decline in their health. So I think this discussion needs to acknowledge all of the data.

Lastly, I want to point something out that I think is critical to understand with regard to my experiences. Brain retraining has *only* been helpful to me in the context of continued and very careful mold avoidance. Brain retraining has in no way replaced mold avoidance, or even come at all close to being a substitute for it. Instead, mold avoidance has absolutely been the foundation of my healing progress. So, all of the above observations should be understood in this light. Even now, after doing over a year of mold avoidance and detox, if I visit buildings or outdoor regions with particularly bad mold toxins, all of this goes out the window. For me, mold exposures are like rat poison. It does not matter what I do with my brain, if I am exposed to rat poison, I get sick. Brain retraining and neuroplasticity are interesting topics, but they won't help the inmate on death row who is being euthanized. And in fact, brain retraining can really hurt people who are being exposed to damaging mycotoxins and are trying to train themselves to ignore these exposures. Just like it would be crazy for someone getting a third degree burn to train themselves to ignore the pain and continue being burned.

One final comment. Some mold avoiders who have pursued extreme avoidance for an extended period of time, later say that they started brain retraining and then credit brain retraining with their healing. I think this is an extremely misleading position. It would be like a person with a broken leg who has been in a cast healing for 6 months, to credit their healing with the Coca Cola they drank last night, ignoring the 6 months of recovery they've been undergoing in the cast. It is easy to overlook this, and not realize what *actually* caused the healing. Even if brain retraining does seem to "do something," I still definitely credit mold avoidance with building up my system to the point where it is strong enough to handle more exposures. Brain retraining has been nothing more than a small side show for me. In fact, I'm pretty sure I would not even be alive if it were not for the 15 months of extreme mold avoidance I've done, and I DID try brain retraining approaches early on. I'm not just sharing my "philosophy" here. I'm sharing what has actually happened to me.

Mold avoidance has literally resurrected me from the dead. It is upsetting to me that some people who are extremely ill may overlook mold avoidance because they do not understand how dangerous these toxins actually are. Please carefully consider this, and do your own research on the damage that mycotoxins can cause.

As usual, I want you to understand that I'm not claiming that my observations are absolutely applicable to everyone. I'm only sharing with you what I've experienced. In no way do I pretend that I have all the answers here. I am eagerly awaiting further science and data on these topics. But I do hope that my observations have been helpful to you, in navigating this topic for yourself. Please do your own research and rely on other resources before coming to conclusions about this topic.

Chapter 27

MOLD IS WEIRD

I would like to conclude this book by telling you that mold is weird. Mold is weird! I'm going to keep saying it until you get it. Didn't hear me? Mold is weird.

No, I'm not a 3rd grader using third grade language. Mold actually IS weird, and it is only when you understand this that mold avoidance starts to make sense. This is important!

Even after over a year of mold avoidance, I struggled to "get it." I wanted to think that mold is similar to other toxins. Toxins that behave normally as you would expect them to. But mold is weird. Do you need to hear it again? Mold is weird.

A mold avoider I know called mold a "pulsating electronic blob." Studies have shown that a certain type of mold called slime mold is made up of millions of independent, seemingly not living, cells, which, when they come together, form a massive blob with a collective consciousness and intelligence. This blob has no central nervous system or brain (after all, it is comprised of many identical independent cells), yet the blob shows signs of intelligence and decision-making, and it operates in unison as one large organism. It even remembers things that researchers taught it, and the memory doesn't fade after a whole year. Is that weird?

Mold is weird.

Mold also seems to behave like a magnet, being attracted to mold sick people. This observation is consistent across many mold avoiders. It is possible that the mold already inside of us, or, some infection inside of us, attracts the mold to itself, causing a sort of locus of effect.

When we get environmental mold hits, such as watching a movie in a moldy theatre, how are these hits hurting us? Is the mold that contaminates our skin somehow entering the body and joining forces with the blob already inside of us? Is the blob living or dead? Does that question even apply to mold in the same way that it applies to other life? Is the mold inside us communicating with the mold outside of us, in the environment?

Science doesn't fully understand mold. Mold is weird. How mold makes us ill and how to recover from mold is also not fully understood, and is weird. Stay with me here, I'm taking you someplace important.

In extreme mold avoidance, if you think of mold as not being weird, then you are missing the path. Because mold is weird, mold avoidance and mold detox is weird. It is different from many of the normal therapies Lyme sufferers are used to. Think of mold as a sticky, mysterious, pulsating, magnetic blob. I'm not claiming that this is the scientific definition of mold. But while scientists take the next few decades to figure it out, this is the loose framework that is helpful in understanding mold and mold avoidance.

I'm not a leading scientist in mold study. But what I've learned, is that I don't have to be. Understanding that mold is weird, and learning from the experience and wisdom of those who have done this before, is what matters.

Accepting the weirdness and allowing yourself to learn a new paradigm of healing and detox will give you the flexibility you need to succeed in mold avoidance. The instructions on getting well are already written, and although they are not perfect, at least for me, they were not the limiting factor in my recovery. For me, the limiting factor was accepting that mold is weird and that the recovery process from mold illness is also weird. Only after I accepted this did I start to really follow the path, and appreciate the work of those mold avoiders who have gone before me.

For a long time, I privately debated with myself whether the setbacks I had throughout mold avoidance were due to infectious flare ups or mold toxicity accumulating in my body. While the infectious flare ups certainly did happen and needed to be addressed, I missed the fact that mold toxicity was also building up inside me, because I didn't recognize that mold was weird.

In January, 2019, we were staying at a wonderful state park in New Mexico, a place known to be very healing to people with mold illness. I was in the midst of a setback, feeling not so great. In my mind I was wondering why I was feeling bad. Was it infections flaring up, or was it mold toxicity? Was the mold alive inside my body? It felt weird.

This state park is a campground which encircles a huge, majestic boulder field. I went on a walk one morning through the boulders, and I ended up leaning against a boulder which was being warmed by the sun. It was a cold morning and we were dry camping in our RV, so I was cold. The warmth felt wonderful.

This state park is in New Mexico, a state that is mostly in the middle of nowhere by USA standards. And this campground itself is in the middle of nowhere even by New Mexico's standards. And this boulder field was in the middle of nowhere inside the campground. So I was in the absolute center of nowhere, literally. It is here that I had one of my greatest revelations about mold.

Leaning against this sunny boulder felt very healing. When I lifted up my shirt and leaned my bare back against the boulder, I could feel mold draining out of my nervous system, possibly due to the grounding effects of this boulder.

Putting my hands on the boulder seemed to have the opposite effect, and seemed to cause mold to enter my nervous system. Why? I don't know. Maybe because the mold was traveling along my spine to get to my hands on its way out of my body, and this temporarily increased the mold concentration in my nervous system. And maybe leaning against the boulder with only my back had the opposite effect.

But none of this is the point. The point is that this was only one of many weird things about mold, because mold is weird.

Leaning against this warm boulder with my bare skin on it made me feel good. Really good, like better than any treatment. Mold toxicity seems to be some kind of electrical blob that interacts with nature in weird ways. It can feel like an infection sometimes, and even trick Lyme-sick people into thinking that their main problem is infections, when in fact their main problem is mold toxicity.

When I was walking back to my RV, that's when it happened. The weirdest thing ever. I was no longer grounded to that boulder. I had my shoes on. As I walked back, I could literally feel the mold toxicity that hadn't yet left my body, flowing back UP my body and back into my head, where it resumed causing the misery that mold causes. Whatever problem in my brain that caused mold to be attracted to my brain like a magnet – whether an infection or mold toxicity itself in my brain – seemed to now be pulling the mold back into my brain, literally. Whatever magnetic force that the boulder was exerting to pull the mold away from me, had now been lost, and so the mold went back to my brain.

You can't even imagine how weird this felt. If you are wondering how I could possibly discern this, trust me, when you've been doing extreme mold avoidance for a long time, you become very tuned into what is happening with mold inside your body. Just ask any mold avoider.

Understanding that mold is weird, even if you don't have all the answers, is, in my experience, the most important first step to being able to see why we do what we do in mold avoidance. When you read Lisa and Erik's books, you'll see that mold avoidance is weird. Why do we need to shower after mold hits? Why do even tiny amounts of mold in our environment need to be avoided? Why will the body refuse to detox unless it is in a clear enough environment? Why does mold on our skin seem to be even more important than mold that we ingest? Why does taking a break from mold "unmask" us to the presence of mold in our living environment?

Again, I'm not saying I have all the answers. But accepting the weirdness of mold helped me tremendously in learning and benefiting from mold avoidance. I believe the weirdness of mold is what is keeping many people sick, and many doctors and researchers from understanding this illness. A whole new paradigm is required in order to understand and heal from mold illness.

I believe that Erik and Lisa are way ahead of their times, trailblazers in making sense of this phenomenon.

Why is this stuff important? This is "Lyme Disease Supercharge," a strategy for healing from Lyme disease when all else fails!

While I did get a lot of benefit from ten pass ozone, live bee venom therapy, and, of course, the numerous therapies I've discussed in my past books, the mold "phenomenon" is definitely a deeper layer of illness and healing. Until this layer is uncovered and dealt with, the true cause of this illness will remain uninhibited.

So, in closing, I would like to thank you for taking the time to read "Lyme Disease Supercharge," and I hope that I have helped you to make sense of this illness phenomenon, just as Lisa and Erik have helped me to make sense of it. And I wish you healing and prosperity in your recovery!

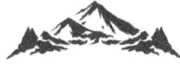

Epilogue

REPORTING FROM THE FRONT LINES

Every author faces the same dilemma: do we hold onto our books endlessly, and wait to publish them until they are perfect? Or, do we release our books into the world when they haven't yet been perfected?

Of course, no book is perfect. So the dilemma is really about knowing when a particular book is "good enough." Which no book ever is, at least in the eyes of the author.

But with this book (the 6th book I've written), this situation was even harder. Because I wrote this book inside of an RV where 5 people are living, not in my usual home office. I miss my home office!

What ended up happening, was that I kept delaying publication of this book, month after month, hoping that I would be able to sit down and make it "more perfect." Only, this never happened. The small tweaks I was working here and there didn't seem to actually be making the book any better. So I finally made the decision to just put the book out into the world. In my opinion, it is an important book. And, it couldn't have been written any other way. Had I written it from my home office, it may have been more polished and perfected, but it would have also been much less insightful. So I prefer to look at this book as the authentic play-by-play journal of a soldier on the front lines of battle, rather than a polished work of literature written by the commander in the comfort of his barracks, far away from the front lines. In other words, there is just no other way this book could have been written and still have offered the value that it offers.

My writing colleague and fellow author, Connie Strasheim, sent me a wonderful list of comments and questions about my book on the eve of the publication date. As I read her comments, I realized that they really needed to be addressed and answered. Yet, I knew that doing so, in book format, would have delayed the release of this book for many more months, due to our RV lifestyle. I felt that there were a lot of people who needed this information, and who wouldn't be getting it soon enough, if I delayed any longer.

So what I have decided to do is to continue the conversation about mold avoidance on my blog, located at www.antilyme.com. Here, I'll respond to Connie's questions and comments. I'll probably create some type of audio file or podcast where I can provide updates and answer questions. I hope to see you over on my blog!

While my book doesn't answer all of the questions, it is a starting point. I hope that it has challenged you to think about chronic illness in new ways.

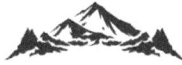

Appendices

These appendices are a collection of posts I've made on the Facebook Mold Avoider's group. I feel that reading them may be informative and educational, but realize that they are written in an informal, conversational style. They are rough and unedited thoughts and observations, so understand them as such.

MOLD IS WEIRD, CONTINUED

Healing from mold is so weird. Mold changed my personality, it drugged me and made me feel like a different person. I sort of got used to that other person. That person had pros and cons, but I got used to him, and that was the new "me." Now, the old me is trying to come back. But it is kind of surprising and I was so used to the other me, that I'm not sure I even want this old me. He is from the past, not the present. How do I become a past person? So weird.

WHO AM I?

In my moldy house, i often got strong flashbacks to the prior house that wasn't moldy. Like I'd wake up and feel like I was in that good house.

I have also had weird flashbacks to the place I went to college.

But lately, in my healing now, the flashbacks are stronger and more vivid than ever.

Also, on my road trip, I am positive that the mycotoxins coming out of me were making me high and delusional, like a drug trip.

So there are all these different "me's."

The me on the road trip. When I'm not exposed, I look back at the road trip me and think ... who was that guy, why were you driving around the desert.

But when I get hits, all of a sudden I'm that road trip guy again.

Then when I'm most clear, I have these intense wacky Tahoe flashbacks. But I can't go to tahoe anymore. So is that the real me?

I feel like that song, "Will the real slim shady please stand up."

This is a big emotional struggle for me. I literally feel like the wiring in my brain is all whacked out. And let me be clear. This is NOT about brain training, because any of these "me's" still react to mold badly. It's more of a physiological brain healing phenomenon.

But I feel sort of displaced. The personality and perspective that makes me who I am, is in flux and I don't know which one to latch onto as the real me.

Can anyone relate to this?

When I'm the most clear, I often don't even want to be on mold avoider forum. But when I'm a little moldy, I love this place and the support and friendships.

So which one is the real me? The one that loves all you guys or the one that wants to move on from this forum?

I literally feel like my stream of consciousness is in flux, and I don't know which part to latch onto as "reality."

Have any of you seen the movie Inception? Where an idea is planted in the brain in a dream, and when they wake up they can't tell what's reality and what's a dream? I FULL ON feel that way.

I think it's made more difficult by the fact that the healthier me, the earlier me, the decades ago me that lived in Tahoe... that's probably the "real " me but I can't go back to Tahoe. But the road trip me was high on mycotoxin detox and doesn't feel like me either. So I'm kind of feeling stuck in purgatory, aka Reno, where I'm not quite either person.

Help!?

PARASITES

I continue to feel that parasites are connected to this illness in all kinds of weird way.

And that other infections like lyme and bartonella really aren't that important, except that they are opportunistic and need to be dealt with.

But when I take parasite Meds, it feels like I'm getting a mold hit. There's some fishy stuff between parasites and mold.

Something fishy... or should I say something moldy... is going on . . .

Emf hits are starting to feel like mold hits... and even parasite drugs are now starting to feel like mold hits . . .

Seems like all of this points back to mold one way or another.

Or, to add a twist into this... maybe mold hits and emf hits are starting to feel like parasites??

Whichever one came first, the chicken or the egg, they sure are interconnected on some deep and spooky level.

MANAGING LIFE IN CIVILIZATION

I think if I couldn't live in a good area, my plan would be to load up my bike, go sleep in my truck illegally in a clear place at a Mtn bike trail head, wake up in the morning clear, then go on a mtn bike ride in a good area while fasted, then show up back into town to live life. This would give me sleep and exercise in a good area. This will be my backup plan I think.

TAHOE/TRUCKEE MOLD

The tahoe / truckee stuff is a whooooooole different ballgame. It's like 100x more dangerous than pretty much anywhere else I've been. Oceanside had lots of Mt, but truckee today put that to shame. Tahoe / truckee is like the North Korea of dangerous places.

Each minute up there is about the same as an hour of a normal mold hit.

THE BLESSINGS OF MOLD AVOIDANCE

I'm actually grateful to be a mold avoider. Even though it is hard as hell and full of challenges.

See, for years, when we were living in our bad house, any therapy I tried was like "meh." "That helped a little maybe?"

But with mold. It's different. It's a bingo.

It feels nice to have a bingo, even if it is a pain. It's motion in the right direction.

Today, went in Home Depot. Not much reaction to chemicals. Nope, that's not it.

Not much reaction to anti-microbials, tho of course they are necessary to keep me stable and moving forward at times.

But in Truckee I didn't even go inside. Just 2 hours in the outdoor air was enough to make me want to die. Bingo. Mt.

Back at my trailer up high in a safe place, I decontaminate... shower. As I'm rubbing off the arms and legs I can feel the mold toxins cleaning away. It's like the stuff is bonded to my skin with glue. Takes a number of washes. With each wash, I'm moaning in contentment and pleasure as my body says more more more. I can feel detox turn back on and my organs start to function. The body as Erik says just would rather store this stuff instead of detoxing it if there's too much of it. It's that dangerous. So as I clear my skin, the body feels safe again to go for it.

This is such a huge bingo or bulls eye.

This is a direction that matters, that makes a huge difference. I'm so grateful for that. As dr dan said to me today, the chaos and disturbance of mold avoidance is still so much better than being sick and debilitated.

Now out of the shower and on my couch listening to the crickets way above Reno on some remote land where all is clear, I can feel my skin burning as if poison ivy had just been washed off. It's burning with pleasure but also feels like a post injury. Erik is right that this stuff is like tear gas. I feel like I could even take another shower and get the last molecules off and that would be worth it, though of course, my 6 gallon trailer water heater is done for tonight.

I'm grateful that this is an answer. It's such a freaking glaring, definitive answer.

GETTING OUTSIDE EVEN WHEN YOU DON'T FEEL LIKE IT

Erik is right!

Was dragging today, just generally off the power curve. Forced myself to go on a bike ride. Then just kept going bigger and longer on the ride. Now, hours later, I feel so much better. Reactivity way down. Mood, energy, focus, optimism way up.

I love that my "prescription" isn't hospitals and surgery and doctors offices. No, it's mountain biking in the beautiful Sierra Nevada mountains. Sometimes when you feel your worst, that's the time to get out of your house or bed and go outside.

WHAT PRISTINE FEELS LIKE

Brandy asked me what pristine feels like to me so I thought my response may interest other group members. This is of course just my observation.

What pristine feels like

That's a great question.

> ❖ my detox pathways turn on like a waterfall, even sometimes making me feel worse and has created scary detox issues, but all the while I feel better somehow. Bile starts flowing like crazy, bile coated stools etc.

> ❖ sugar cravings as the infections get stirred up due to the detox. Then, later in the recovery process, pristine air triggers sugar cravings to completely disappear.

> ❖ elevation doesn't affect me at all, and I can do herculean exercise and feel energized and great. I mean this is so pronounced. I can do bike rides at 9,000 feet like an elite athlete.

> ❖ molds in the area and even buildings don't bother me, and even have a pleasant earthy aroma, like they are 100% natural.

❖ contamination on my own stuff doesn't bother me near as much, because I leap up the power curve so much.

❖ my mental outlook becomes very clear, thinking is clear, problems I had before coming don't seem to daunting anymore, everything seems right with the world.

❖ BONUS POINTS: the best 2 areas near Reno that I have found are also untouched by chemicals. Example- there's this one forest that feels ok but it is national forest and they spray it, but once you cross over into the wilderness area where it isn't managed forest, it's like walking into another world in 200 feet. More animals, oily thriving plants, bugs, earthy smells, spiderwebs everywhere. It is this aspect of "pristine" that I have found to be super important ... when I'm in this zone I can literally feel the microbiome of the wilderness doing battle and killing badness inside me. Literally makes me herx just like ozone would. And I want to stay and never want to leave. It's that different just crossing over from NFS (national forest service) to Wilderness. This is lacking sadly in many camping areas where moldies visit because most camping is NFS. I didn't encounter this at all on our 10,000 mile road trip. You can search for another recent post I made where I posted pics of a bike ride crossing over into Wilderness and my observations.

❖ probably because of the above, when I take a breath, it's a deep relaxing satisfying breath filled with rich earthy aroma, and it is almost euphoric. I used to think I felt this in NFS but now realize it is laced with toxins and only in true wilderness do I feel this.

❖ last sign of pristine for me is when I come back to "town" I feel my oxygen cranking and feel good, have plans for the week, life is in balance, but wham, as soon as I get hit with normal civilization, I tank hard. The wilderness opened up my systems and as Lisa has said when systems are open they are more vulnerable to damage from civilization. So this is another "sign" for me that I was just in a good location.

ON THE LOCATIONS EFFECT

Huge location's effect today. Stumbled into it.

I'm in the middle of a long bike ride in Reno and I am within eyesight of the summit connecting incline.

I'm sorry to say, I can feel wisps of the Tahoe crap in the air (!!!!) and even more bothersome and sad, this beautiful pine forest just feels "off" — it feels like the biome has been erased and replaced with a thin coat of mt.

Which is interesting because it SHOULD be the same biome as my pristine campground – but it's not. Which confirms what Lisa has said that the pristine campground isn't just a LACK of toxins but a PRESENCE of good things. I've been wondering if I should bathe and eat the dirt up there.

And on a similar vein, since taking two diflucan pills MY OWN microbiome has also changed for the worse, as Lisa predicted it might, my body odor is different almost like rotten cheese and I feel different. Which shows to me there really is a colonization issue going on here and these organism are competing for the front runner position. I don't like the winners so i think it's time to go do a "reset" with ten pass then as Lisa suggested maybe go camp in my pristine biome.

Some of this stuff seems like such fiction until you start putting the pieces together. Our bodies are just giant Petri dishes with all these bugs vying for their position. It's still weird to me though that healthy people can do ten pass ozone and nothing happens.

I decided to ride up higher in the mountains and across the national forest boundary. Fascinating. Almost instantly, a healthy microbiome returned. Suspicious that it would be so instant. Logging and chemicals used on the non protected portion? Seems sinister. But also maybe more to it than just Tahoe being nearby. The wilderness space also seems much more densely grown with trees.

In this good biome I can feel the air instantly doing battle against the bad bugs in my sinus, body, almost more powerful than a ozone sinus treatment (!!!!!!). Which makes me think our "good" locations are more about the addition of than subtraction of stuff.

Also... with this experience I can't help but wonder why Erik would question the need to leave an entire region. To me, almost all of Tahoe feels bad, like that same tainted and devoid biome, even areas where Mt isn't actively present — because maybe the Mt was present ENOUGH during storms and wind to wipe out the biome.

In this good space the plants are more vibrant and oily, there are more bugs and spider webs and there's a weird organic earthy odor. I mean it's wild. Feels like lord of the rings or Peter Pan. Smells, animals, critters, everywhere.

Also. This makes me feel like emf isn't the whole game. Emf wouldn't seem to shut off instantly.

It may be just as good as my pristine campground!

This seems like a secondary benefit of the famous "hiking to elevation." That is, biome.

MORE ON THE IMPORTANCE OF GETTING OUTSIDE

When I woke up this morning I was dragging but remember Erik saying "that's when you need to go."

By the time I had ridden from 6000 to 7500 feet I began to turn into Superman. And wanted to keep going but need to plan better. And someone said mountain lions.

So today was a fascinating day. 3 Biomes in one day. Pristine, not so great forest, and Great Basin reno. And while on a bike with blood vessels open, more vivid perceptions. Reno itself really is yucky now that I'm back but the time in pristine air does help I think . . .

It's also interesting to note that on our road trip I rarely found these opportunities. Not enough elevation most places and a lot of private property. So booo for Reno being yucky but yay for it having two pristine spots I've found now.

I don't mind sharing where this one is, most but for the fittest of us will never make it up there. The first half of the trail is not pristine. It's a long haul on rough terrain to get to the good stuff.

Seems so important to heal and push to the point that the body can do this stuff, it's like a tipping point. When I was the most mold sick, I couldn't really hike and exercise. I feel like that was the turning point of becoming super-sick.

I still think I'm going to need to get ozone though.

I did rub some dirt and plants on me up there. Some of it felt good. One of them felt really bad. But I do think the air and being immersed in the biome is the key

I can't describe how dramatic the change was and how much it energized and recharged me. Mind blowing.

BIOME TOUR

Has anyone else craved a "biome tour" as they recover?

For a long time I craved the tahoe hometown biome. But now, for some reason, I've been having visions of and intense cravings to go back to my college town biome where I started getting sick. It is on my way home so I'm considering it.

But is this a craving to be indulged or is it just some random brain misfire?

Perhaps our body's really do want us to travel through multiple regions and cities, as a way to repopulate our flora by breathing different air. Like probiotics in the air. This is actually a scientifically proven phenomenon.

ARIZONA LOCATION OBSERVATIONS

Had an interesting day "perceptifying".

Had to drive 100 miles rt to thatcher today. Amazing how you can just feel the MT plumes.

Turns out our beloved dragoon going bad is a combination of factors to the best of my knowledge.

❖ junk from Tucson is now blowing in here all the way to 5 mi east of wilcox. I think the rain and wind increased the amount of junk and how far it traveled.

❖ the sewer and buildings on our property... Same story. Rain and cold brought stuff out.

❖ all the toxins now are magnified because of the relative shift phenomenon.

Everyone felt the plume slam us like a brick wall driving back west on the 10. Wife and son too. It's amazing how when air goes bad we often are in disbelief and blame it on other things like just general health declining when in fact it is the air. Very surreal.

It's even more apparent now how bad it is having had a 1 day Sabbatical from this place. For the last week I've been unable to even muster the attention to get work done on my laptop and I've not even cared – mold apathy. But on the road today away, I had all this motivation and clarity and started getting the "sausage fingers" sign of pristine air, again.

I can also see now why traveling around a lot is really the only way to learn mold avoidance, because the shifts are so subtle and unbelievable that you'd never recognize them let alone believe them unless you have personally experienced them many times.

HUMOR OF MOLD AVOIDER LIFE

If people are gonna walk by and gawk and judge me when I'm getting out of sleeping in my truck for the night, note to self, it's better for them to see me when I'm half way out of the tailgate, cuz then I can pretend I'm just leaning inside to get something. Duly noted. LOL

#moldavoiderlife

Also, I think it's funny that I now openly walk around campgrounds in my boxers. It's like my livingroom. Ha!

PARASITES AND FENBENDAZOLE

(Disclaimer: fenbendazole is a drug which is not approved for human consumption. I do not recommend that people take this drug).

Took some fenbendazole. Oh my gosh. Strongest single herx event I've ever had. Also had about an hour of feeling more clear than I've felt in 20 years. It seemed to be hitting really deep stuff that never gets hit effectively. It was so strong that I was having flashbacks to many pre-sick moments all night. Like I'd wake up throughout the night and wonder why I was in an rv; having flashbacks like it's time to get ready to go to work (to a job I had 20 years ago). Who knows if any improvements will be long term.

LIVING OUTDOORS FOR AN ENTIRE SUMMER

I've been living outside all summer. Literally, outside, all summer. The truth is stranger than fiction. Right now pretty much my only indoor safe place this summer in the heat, is the Burger King inside walmart. No mold, good a/c to keep cool, table to work at. Trailer is contaminated and apartment has EMF. Wish I could move my family in here. So, if I don't want to be outside, and I want to feel OK, I can be sleeping in the back of my truck or at Walmart :/

A CAUTIONARY TALE ON WATER

So we arrived at city of rocks about 2 weeks ago. Air fantastic, lots of healing. But mysteriously I started going downhill.

I began to suspect the water. It felt like that Erik story of water being worst after clothing DRIES, cyano bacteria. But there also felt to be some x-factor in the water, maybe copper or some radioactive contaminant.

But the water was everywhere...we had already done some laundry, washed bedding, and I had showered in it.
So we drove 300 miles to a different campground, to try to find a good walmart and do laundry. It sort of didn't work out, and I was still getting worse.

So we drove back 300 miles to City of Rocks, because the air is good here and I still think air is much harder to hack than water.

So I made an attempt to get away from this water while being here, but it was kind of half-baked attempt. I kept not doing well.

So last night I woke up in the middle of the night, and I was like, "Bryan, you need to kick ass tomorrow and get this done, no matter how you feel."

So I woke up, we had 9 one gallon crystal gueser's left. I rationed them – some for laundry, some to drink, some to wash bedding, some for a shower.

If you are doing the math, you'll see that the water had to go a LOOONG way. My wife won't be going back to Walmart until tomorrow, and since its a 40 minute drive and she has to decontaminate when she returns, I didn't want to make her go today.

Long story short, after making a COMPLETE break with the water here.... all new clothing ($20 at walmart), ditching the sleeping bag I washed in the water, a new fleece blanket washed in bottled water, and a shower in bottled water (2 gallons will do it... I've become very efficient, despite being quite hairy).... I am FINALLY feeling back to my old self, after 2 weeks of torment. This water really snuck up on me here, and if we ever come back next Winter, I'll be sure to plan ahead for the water issues.

Boiling the water here MIGHT have worked but I was in dire straights and needed a sure solution, so I opted for bottled water for everything.

My family has been drinking the water here – gulp?? – and Ellen said she didn't have a problem with the water, so maybe it is an individual thing and/or seasonal. My son has been feeling ill so tomorrow we'll switch all people to drinking bottled water.

Anyway, this was just a crazy two weeks. I really have learned the value of minimalism. I guess it has become my goal to be able to survive anywhere on ten crystal guesser water bottles for – laundry, drinking, showering, and washing bedding. Obviously that isn't a long-term solution – to constantly be using bottled water... but it's good to be able to do in an emergency. And I like John's thoughts on turning up the furnace instead of needing a warm sleeping bag – propane is much easier to come by right now than a good sleeping bag.

Anyway, folks, watch out for your water! It could be keeping you sick!

And as a note.... I'm NOT a water snob or usually affected by water. I'd say only 2 or 3 of our 60+ stops have had issues like this. In Anaheim, the water is totally fine for me and I shower in it and do great. So I'm not sure what it is about THIS water, but it sure is kryptonite to me.

Happy Hydration!

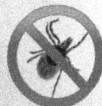

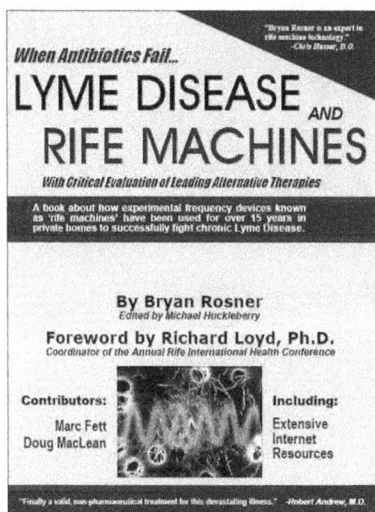

By Bryan Rosner
Edited by Michael Huckleberry

Foreword by Richard Loyd, Ph.D.
Coordinator of the Annual Rife International Health Conference

Contributors:
Marc Fett
Doug MacLean

Including:
Extensive
Internet
Resources

"Finally a valid, non-pharmaceutical treatment for this devastating illness." -Robert Andrew, M.D.

Book • $35

When Antibiotics Fail: Lyme Disease And Rife Machines, With Critical Evaluation Of Leading Alternative Therapies

By Bryan Rosner
Foreword by Richard Loyd, Ph.D.

There are enough books and websites about what Lyme disease is and which ticks carry it. But there is very little useful information for people who actually have a case of Lyme disease that is not responding to conventional antibiotic treatment. Lyme disease sufferers need to know their options, not how to identify a tick.

This book describes how experimental electromagnetic frequency devices known as rife machines have been used for over 15 years in private homes to fight Lyme disease. Also included are evaluations of more than 25 conventional and alternative Lyme disease therapies, including:

- Homeopathy
- IV and oral antibiotics
- Mercury detox.
- Hyperthermia / saunas
- Ozone and oxygen
- Samento®
- Colloidal Silver
- Bacterial die-off detox.

- Colostrum
- Magnesium supplementation
- Hyperbaric oxygen chamber (HBOC)
- ICHT Italian treatment
- Non-pharmaceutical antibiotics
- Exercise, diet and candida protocols
- Cyst-targeting antibiotics
- The Marshall Protocol®

Many Lyme disease sufferers have heard of rife machines, some have used them. But until now, there has not been a concise and organized source to explain how and why they have been used by Lyme patients. In fact, this is the first book ever published on this important topic.

The Foreword for the book is by Richard Loyd, Ph.D., coordinator of the annual Rife International Health Conference. The book takes a practical, down-to-earth approach which allows you to learn about*:

"This book provides life-saving insights for Lyme disease patients."

- Richard Loyd, Ph.D.

- Antibiotic treatment problems and shortcomings—why some people choose to use rife machines after other therapies fail.
- Hypothetical treatment schedules and sessions, based on the author's experience.
- The experimental machines with the longest track record: High Power Magnetic Pulser, EMEM Machine, Coil Machine, and AC Contact Machine.
- Explanation of the "herx reaction" and why it may indicate progress.
- The intriguing story that led to the use of rife machines to fight Lyme disease 20 years ago.
- Antibiotic categories and classifications, with pros and cons of each type of drug.
- Visit our website to read FREE EXCERPTS from the book!

Disclaimer: *Your treatment decisions must be made under the care of a licensed physician. Rife machines are not FDA approved and the FDA has not reviewed or approved of these books. The author is a layperson, not a doctor, and much of the content of these books is a statement of opinion based on the author's personal experience and research.*

Paperback book, 8.5 x 11", 203 pages, $35

The Top 10 Lyme Disease Treatments: Defeat Lyme Disease With The Best Of Conventional And Alternative Medicine

By Bryan Rosner
Foreword by James Schaller, M.D.

This information-packed book identifies ten promising conventional and alternative Lyme disease treatments and gives practical guidance on integrating them into a comprehensive treatment plan that you and your physician can customize for your individual situation and needs.

The book was not written to replace Bryan Rosner's first book (*Lyme Disease and Rife Machines*, opposing page). It was written to complement that book, offering Lyme sufferers many new foundational and supportive treatment options, based on the author's extensive research and years of personal experience. Topics include*:

Book • $35

- Systemic enzyme therapy, which helps detoxify tissues and blood, reduce inflammation, stimulate the immune system, and kill Lyme disease bacteria.
- Lithium orotate, a powerful yet all-natural mineral (belonging to the same mineral group as sodium and potassium) capable of profound neuroprotective activity.
- Thorough and extensive coverage of a complete Lyme disease detoxification program, including discussion of both liver and skin detoxification pathways. Specific detoxification therapies such as liver cleanses, bowel cleanses, the Shoemaker Neurotoxin Elimination Protocol, sauna therapy, mineral baths, mineral supplementation, milk thistle, and many others. Ideas to reduce and control herx reactions.
- Tips and clinical research from James Schaller, M.D.
- A detailed look at one method for utilizing antibiotics during a rife machine treatment campaign.
- Wide coverage of the Marshall Protocol, including an in-depth discussion of its mechanism of action in relation to Lyme disease pathology. Also, the author's personal experience with the Marshall Protocol over 3 years.
- An explanation of and new information about the Salt / Vitamin C protocol.
- Hot-off-the-press information on mangosteen fruit (not to be confused with mango) and its many benefits, including antibacterial, anti-inflammatory, and anti-cancer properties.
- New guidelines for combining all the therapies discussed in both of Rosner's books into a complete treatment plan. Brief and articulate for consideration by you and your doctor.
- Also includes updates on rife therapy, cutting-edge supplements, political challenges, an exclusive interview with Willy Burgdorfer, Ph.D. (discoverer of Lyme), and much more!

"Bryan Rosner thinks big and this new book offers big solutions."
- James Schaller, M.D.

"Another ground-breaking Lyme Disease book."
- Jeff Mittelman, moderator of the Lyme-and-rife group

"Brilliant and thorough."
- Nenah Sylver, Ph.D.

Do not miss this top Lyme disease resource. Discover new healing tools today! Bring this book to your doctor's appointment to help with forming a treatment plan.

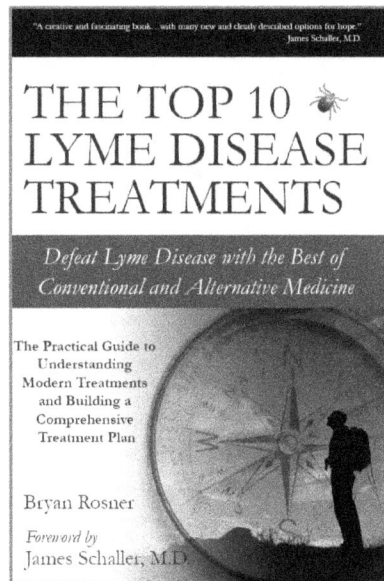

Paperback book, 7 x 10", 367 pages, $35

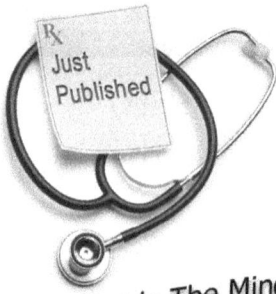

Rx
Just Published

13 Lyme Doctors Share Treatment Strategies!

In this new book, not one, but thirteen Lyme-literate healthcare practitioners describe the tools they use in their practices to heal patients from chronic Lyme disease. Never before available in book format!

Get Inside The Minds Of Top Lyme Doctors!

**Insights Into Lyme Disease Treatment:
13 Lyme Literate Health Care Practitioners
Share Their Healing Strategies**

By Connie Strasheim
Foreword by Maureen Mcshane, M.D.

If you traveled the country for appointments with 13 Lyme-literate health care practitioners, you would discover many cutting-edge therapies used to combat chronic Lyme disease. You would also spend thousands of dollars on hotels, plane tickets, and medical appointment fees—not to mention the time it would take to embark on such a journey.

Even if you had the time and money to travel, would the physicians have enough time to answer all of your questions? Would you even know which questions to ask?

In this long-awaited book, health care journalist and Lyme patient Connie Strasheim

Paperback • 443 Pages • $39.95

has done all the work for you. She conducted intensive interviews with 13 of the world's most competent Lyme disease healers, asking them thoughtful, important questions, and then spent months compiling their information into 13 organized, user-friendly chapters that contain the core principles upon which they base their medical treatment of chronic Lyme disease. The practitioners' backgrounds span a variety of disciplines, including allopathic, naturopathic, complementary, chiropractic, homeopathic, and energy medicine. All aspects of treatment are covered, from anti-microbial remedies and immune system support, to hormonal restoration, detoxification, and dietary/lifestyle choices. **PHYSICIANS INTERVIEWED:**

- Steven Bock, M.D.
- Ginger Savely, DNP
- Ronald Whitmont, M.D.
- Nicola McFadzean, N.D.
- Jeffrey Morrison, M.D.
- Steven J. Harris, M.D.
- Peter J. Muran, M.D., M.B.A.

- Ingo D. E. Woitzel, M.D.
- Susan L. Marra, M.S., N.D.
- W. Lee Cowden, M.D., M.D. (H)
- Deborah Metzger, Ph.D., M.D.
- Marlene Kunold, "Heilpraktiker"
- Elizabeth Hesse-Sheehan, DC, CCN
- Visit our website to read a FREE CHAPTER!

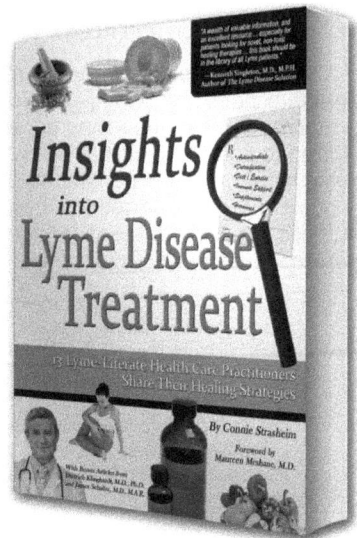

Paperback book, 7 x 10", 443 pages, $39.95

Rife International Health Conference
Feature-Length DVD (93 Minutes)

Bryan Rosner's Presentation and Interview with Doug MacLean

The Official Rife Technology Seminar Seattle, WA, USA

If you have been unable to attend the Rife International Health Conference, this DVD is your opportunity to watch two very important Lyme-related presentations from the event:

DVD • $24.50

Presentation #1: Bryan Rosner's Sunday morning talk entitled *Lyme Disease: New Paradigms in Diagnosis and Treatment - the Myths, the Reality, and the Road Back to Health.* (51 minutes)

Presentation #2: Bryan Rosner's interview with Doug MacLean, in which Doug talked about his experiences with Lyme disease, including the incredible journey he undertook to invent the first modern rife machine used to fight Lyme disease. Although Doug's journey as a Lyme disease pioneer took place 20 years ago, this was the first time Doug has ever accepted an invitation to appear in public. This is the only video available where you can see Doug talk about what it was like to be the first person ever to use rife technology as a treatment for Lyme disease. Now you can see how it all began. Own this DVD and own a piece of history! (42 minutes)

Lymebook.com has secured a special licensing agreement with JS Enterprises, the Canadian producer of the Rife Conference videos, to bring this product to you at the special low price of $24.50. Total DVD viewing time: 1 hour, 33 minutes. We have DVDs in stock, shipped to you within 3 business days.

Price Comparison (should you get the DVD?)

Cost of attending the recent Rife Conference (2 people):
Hotel Room, 3 Nights = $400
Registration = $340
Food = $150
Airfare = $600
Total = $1,490

Cost of the DVD, which you can view as many times as you want, and show to family and friends:
DVD = $24.50

Bryan Rosner Presenting on Sunday Morning In Seattle

**DVD
93 Minutes
$24.50**

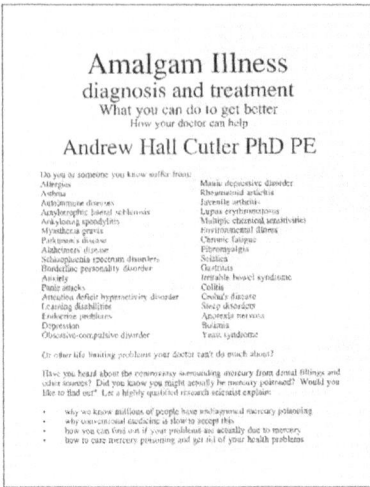

Amalgam Illness

diagnosis and treatment

What you can do to get better
How your doctor can help

Andrew Hall Cutler PhD PE

Do you or someone you know suffer from:

Allergies · Manic depressive disorder
Asthma · Rheumatoid arthritis
Autoimmune diseases · Juvenile arthritis
Amyotrophic lateral sclerosis · Lupus erythematosus
Ankylosing spondylitis · Multiple chemical sensitivities
Myasthenia gravis · Environmental illness
Parkinson's disease · Chronic fatigue
Alzheimer's disease · Fibromyalgia
Schizophrenia spectrum disorders · Sciatica
Borderline personality disorder · Gastritis
Anxiety · Irritable bowel syndrome
Panic attacks · Colitis
Attention deficit hyperactivity disorder · Crohn's disease
Learning disabilities · Sleep disorders
Endocrine problems · Anorexia nervosa
Depression · Bulimia
Obsessive-compulsive disorder · Yeast syndrome

Or other life limiting problems your doctor can't do much about?

Have you heard about the controversy surrounding mercury from dental fillings and other issues? Did you know you might actually be mercury poisoned? Would you like to find out? Let a highly qualified research scientist explain:

· why we know millions of people have undiagnosed mercury poisoning
· why conventional medicine is slow to accept this
· how you can find out if your problems are actually due to mercury
· how to cure mercury poisoning and get rid of your health problems

Book • $35

Amalgam Illness, Diagnosis and Treatment: What You Can Do to Get Better, How Your Doctor Can Help

By Andrew Cutler, PhD

This book was written by a chemical engineer who himself got mercury poisoning from his amalgam dental fillings. He found that there was no suitable educational material for either the patient or the physician. Knowing how much people can suffer from this condition, he wrote this book to help them get well. With a PhD in chemistry from Princeton University and extensive study in biochemistry and medicine, Andrew Cutler uses layman's terms to explain how people become mercury poisoned and what to do about it. The author's research shows that mercury poisoning can easily be cured at home with over-the-counter oral chelators – this book explains how.

In the book you will find practical guidance on how to tell if you really have chronic mercury poisoning or some other problem. Proper diagnostic procedures are provided so that sick people can decide what is wrong rather than trying random treatments. If mercury poisoning is your problem, the book tells you how to get the mercury out of your body, and how to feel good while you do that. The treatment section gives step-by-step directions to figure out exactly what mercury is doing to you and how to fix it.

"Dr. Cutler uses his background in chemistry to explain the safest approach to treat mercury poisoning. I am a physician and am personally using his protocol on myself."

- Melissa Myers, M.D.

Sections also explain how the scientific literature shows many people must be getting poisoned by their amalgam fillings, why such a regulatory blunder occurred, and how the debate between "mainstream" and "alternative" medicine makes it more difficult for you to get the medical help you need.

This down-to-earth book lets patients take care of themselves. It also lets doctors who are not familiar with chronic mercury intoxication treat it. The book is a practical guide to getting well. Sections from the book include:

• Why worry about mercury poisoning?
• What mercury does to you – symptoms, laboratory test irregularities, diagnostic checklist.
• How to treat mercury poisoning easily with oral chelators.
• Dealing with other metals including copper, arsenic, lead, cadmium.
• Dietary and supplement guidelines.
• Balancing hormones during the recovery process.
• How to feel good while you are chelating the metals out.
• How heavy metals cause infections to thrive in the body.
• Politics and mercury.

This is the world's most authoritative, accurate book on mercury poisoning.

Paperback book, 8.5 x 11", 226 pages, $35

Hair Test Interpretation: Finding Hidden Toxicities

By Andrew Cutler, PhD

Hair tests are worth doing because a surprising number of people diagnosed with incurable chronic health conditions actually turn out to have a heavy metal problem; quite often, mercury poisoning. Heavy metal problems can be corrected. Hair testing allows the underlying problem to be identified – and the chronic health condition often disappears with proper detoxification.

Hair Test Interpretation: Finding Hidden Toxicities is a practical book that explains how to interpret **Doctor's Data, Inc.** and **Great Plains Laboratory** hair tests. A step-by-step discussion is provided, with figures to illustrate the process and make it easy. The book gives examples using actual hair test results from real people.

Hair Test Interpretation: Finding Hidden Toxicities

Andrew Hall Cutler, Ph. D., P. E.

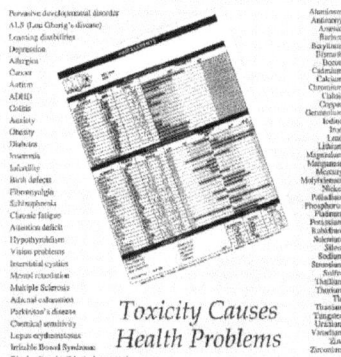

Toxicity Causes Health Problems

Book • $35

One of the problems with hair testing is that both conventional and alternative health care providers do not know how to interpret these tests. Interpretation is not as simple as looking at the results and assuming that any mineral out of the reference range is a problem mineral.

Interpretation is complicated because heavy metal toxicity, especially mercury poisoning, interferes with mineral transport throughout the body. Ironically, if someone is mercury poisoned, hair test mercury is often low and other minerals may be elevated or take on unusual values. For example, mercury often causes retention of arsenic, antimony, tin, titanium, zirconium, and aluminum. An inexperienced health care provider may wrongfully assume that one of these other minerals is the culprit, when in reality mercury is the true toxicity.

"This new book of Andrew's is the definitive guide in the confusing world of heavy metal poisoning diagnosis and treatment. I'm a practicing physician, 20 years now, specializing in detoxification programs for treatment of resistant conditions. It was fairly difficult to diagnose these heavy metal conditions before I met Andrew Cutler and developed a close relationship with him while reading his books. In this book I found his usual painful attention to detail gave a solid framework for understanding the complexity of mercury toxicity as well as the less common exposures. You really couldn't ask for a better reference book on a subject most researchers and physicians are still fumbling in the dark about."
- Dr. Rick Marschall

So, as you can see, getting a hair test is only the first step. The second step is figuring out what the hair test means. Andrew Cutler, PhD, is a registered professional chemical engineer with years of experience in biochemical and healthcare research. This clear and concise book makes hair test interpretation easy, so that you know which toxicities are causing your health problems.

Paperback book, 8.5 x 11", 298 pages, $35

Mold Illness and Mold Remediation Made Simple: Removing Mold Toxins from Bodies and Sick Buildings

By James Schaller, M.D. and Gary Rosen, Ph.D.

Indoor mold toxins are much more dangerous and prevalent than most people realize. Visible mold in and around your house is far less dangerous than the mold you cannot see. Indoor mold toxicity, in addition to causing its own unique set of health problems and symptoms, also greatly contributes to the severity of most chronic illnesses.

In this book, a top physician and experienced contractor team up to help you quickly recover from indoor mold exposure. This book is easy to read with many color photographs and illustrations.

Book • $32.95

Paperback book, 8.5 x 11", 140 pages, $32.95
Also available on our website as an eBook!

Go online to **www.LymeBook.com** to learn more about these new books, just released!

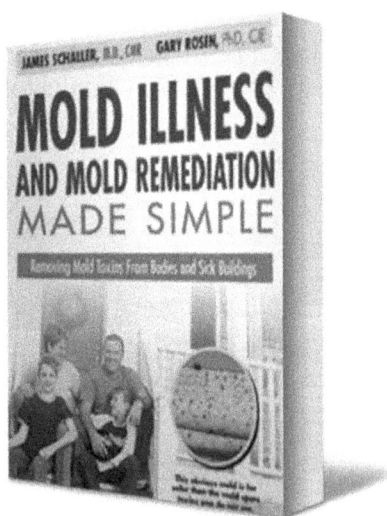

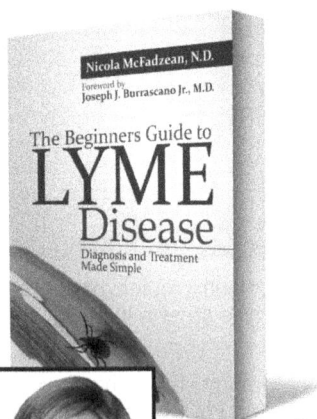

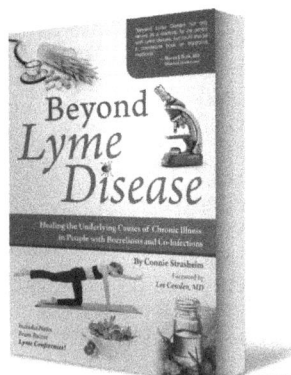

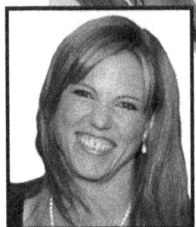

Don't miss these great new resources by authors Connie Strasheim and Nicola McFadzean, ND. Above left: *The Beginner's Guide to Lyme Disease*. Above right: *Beyond Lyme Disease*.

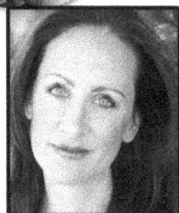

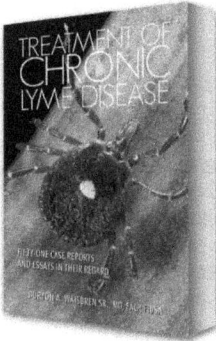

Treatment of Chronic Lyme Disease: 51 Case Reports and Essays In Their Regard

By Burton Waisbren Sr., MD, FACP, FIDSA

DON'T MISS THIS BOOK! A MUST-HAVE RESOURCE. What sets this Lyme disease book apart are the credentials of its author: he is not only a Fellow of the Infectious Diseases Society of America (IDSA), he is also one of its Founders! With 57+ years experience in medicine, Dr. Waisbren passionately argues for the validity of chronic Lyme disease and presents useful information about 51 cases of the disease which he has personally treated. His position is in stark contrast to that of the IDSA, which is a very powerful organization. **Quite possibly the most important book ever published on Lyme disease, as a result of the author's experience and credentials.**

Book • $24.95

Paperback book, 6x9", 169 pages, $24.95

Bartonella:
Diagnosis and Treatment

By James Schaller, M.D.

2 Book Set • $99.95

As an addition to his growing collection of informative books, Dr. James Schaller penned this excellent 2-part volume on Bartonella, a Lyme disease co-infection. The set is an ideal complementary resource to his Babesia textbook (next page).

Bartonella infections occur throughout the entire world, in cities, suburbs, and rural locations. It is found in fleas, dust mites, ticks, lice, flies, cat and dog saliva, and insect feces.

This 2-book set provides advanced treatment strategies as well as detailed diagnostic criteria, with dozens of full-color illustrations and photographs.

Both books in this 2-part set are included with your order.

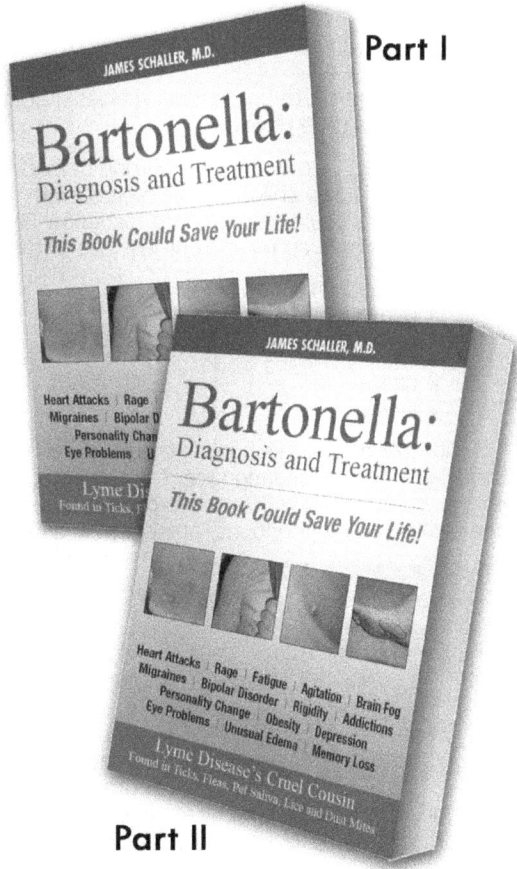

Part I

Part II

2 paperback books included, 7 x 10", 500 pages, $99.95

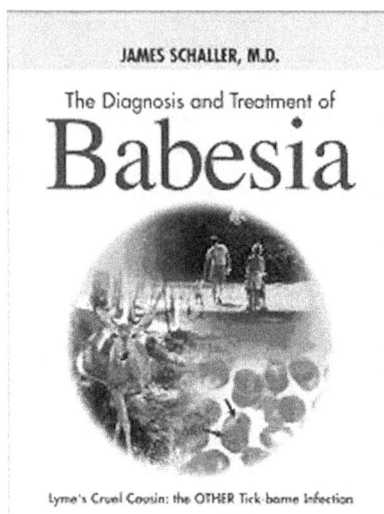

JAMES SCHALLER, M.D.

The Diagnosis and Treatment of

Babesia

Lyme's Cruel Cousin: the OTHER Tick-borne Infection

Book • $55

The Diagnosis and Treatment of Babesia: Lyme's Cruel Cousin – The Other Tick-Borne Infection

By James Schaller, M.D.

Do you or a loved one experience excess fatigue? Have you ever had unusually high fevers, chills, or sweats? You may have Babesia, a very common tick-borne infection. Babesia is often found with Lyme disease and, like all tick-borne infections, is rarely diagnosed and reported accurately.

The deer tick which carries Lyme disease and Babesia may be as small as a poppy seed and injects a painkiller, an antihistamine, and an anticoagulant to avoid detection. As a result, many people have Babesia and do not know it. Numerous forms of Babesia are carried by ticks. This book introduces patients and health care workers to the various species that infect humans and are not routinely tested for by sincere physicians.

Dr. Schaller, who practices medicine in Florida, first became interested in Babesia after one of his own children was infected with it. None of the elite pediatricians or child specialists could help. No one tested for Babesia or considered it a possible diagnosis. His child suffered from just two of these typical Babesia symptoms:

- Significant Fatigue
- Coughing
- Dizziness
- Trouble Thinking
- Fevers
- Memory Loss
- Chills
- Air Hunger
- Headache
- Sweats
- Unresponsiveness to Lyme Treatment

With 374 pages, this book is the most current and comprehensive book on Babesia in the English language. It reviews thousands of articles and presents the results of interviews with world experts on the subject. It offers you top information and broad treatment options, presented in a clear and simple manner. All treatments are explained thoroughly, including their possible side effects, drug interactions, various dosing strategies, pros/cons, and physician experiences.

"Once again Dr. Schaller has provided us with a much-needed and practical resource. This book gave me exactly what I was looking for."

- Thomas W., Patient

Finally, the book also addresses many other aspects of practical medical care often overlooked in this infection, such as treatment options for managing fatigue. Plainly stated, this book is a must-have for patients and health care providers who deal with Lyme disease and its co-infections. Dr. Schaller's many years in clinical practice give the book a practical angle that many other similar books lack. Don't miss this user-friendly resource!

Paperback book, 7 x 10", 374 pages, $55
Also available on our website as an eBook!

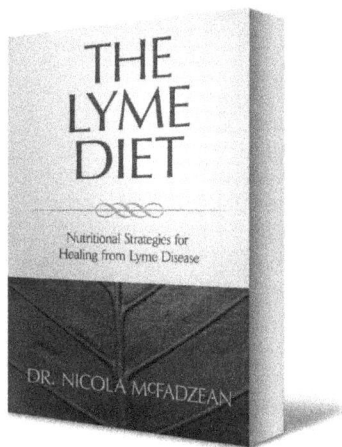

The Lyme Diet: Nutritional Strategies for Healing from Lyme Disease

By Nicola McFadzean, N.D.

We know about antibiotics and herbs. But what is the right diet for Lyme sufferers? Now you can read about the experience of Dr. Nicola McFadzean, N.D., in treating Lyme patients using proper diet.

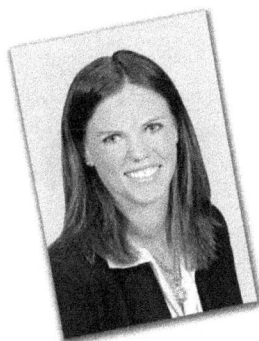

The author is a Naturopathic Doctor and graduate of Bastyr University in Seattle, Washington. She is currently in

Book • $24.95

Nicola McFadzean, N.D.

private practice at her clinic, RestorMedicine, located in San Diego, California.

This book covers numerous topics (not just diet-related):

- Reducing and controlling inflammation
- Maximizing immune function via dietary choices
- Restoring the gut & regaining healthy digestion
- Detoxification with food

- Hormone imbalances
- Biofilms
- Kefir vs. yogurt vs. probiotics
- Candida, liver support, and much more!

Paperback book, 6x9", 214 Pages, $24.95
Also available as an eBook on our website!

Cannabis for Lyme Disease & Related Conditions: Scientific Basis & Anecdotal Evidence for Medicinal Use *By Shelley White, with Foreword by Julie McIntyre, Clinical Herbalist*

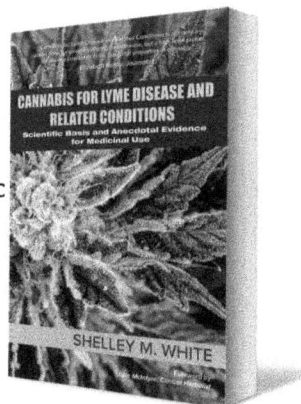

Natural medicine has proven helpful for many Lyme sufferers. Unfortunately, Lyme herbalists and naturopathic doctors are relatively scarce, and treatments can be expensive. It is clear that more practical herbal treatments are in great demand. This book meets that demand, and offers an in-depth and easy-to-understand guide to walk patients through the natural treatment process. White's personal experience treating her own Lyme disease with cannabis, along with her background as a writer and researcher, inspired this book. Readers will find out about various aspects of cannabis and its medicinal uses, including its antibacterial properties, chemical constituents, strains, forms and methods of use, as well as recipes, safety, and legal considerations.

Paperback Book • $24.95

Paperback book, 6x9", 260 pages, $24.95

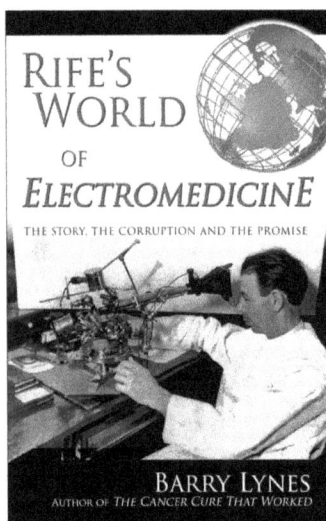

Rife's World of Electromedicine: The Story, the Corruption and the Promise

By Barry Lynes

The cause of cancer was discovered in the early 1930's. It was a virus-sized, mini-bacteria or "particle" that induced cells to become malignant and grow into tumors. The cancer microbe or particle was given the name BX by the brilliant scientist who discovered it: Royal Raymond Rife.

Laboratory verification of the cause of cancer was done hundreds of times with mice in order to be absolutely certain. Five of America's most prominent physicians helped oversee clinical trials managed by a major university's medical school.

Sixteen cancer patients were brought by ambulance twice a week to the clinical trial location in La Jolla, California. There they were treated with a revolutionary electromedicine that painlessly, non-invasively destroyed only the cancer-causing microbe or particle named BX. After just three months of this therapy, all patients were diagnosed as clinically cured. Later, the therapy was suppressed and remains so today.

In 1987, Barry Lynes wrote the classic book on Rife history (*The Cancer Cure That Worked*, see catalog page 14). *Rife's World* is the sequel.

Book • $17.95

Paperback book, 5.5 x 8.5", 90 pages, $17.95

Physicians' Desk Reference (PDR) Books (opposing page)

Most people have heard of *Physicians' Desk Reference* (PDR) books because, for over 60 years, physicians and researchers have turned to PDR for the latest word on prescription drugs.

THOMSON

You may not know that Thomson Healthcare, publisher of PDR, offers PDR reference books not only for drugs, but also for herbal and nutritional supplements. No available books come even close to the amount of information provided in these PDRs—*PDR for Herbal Medicines* weighs 5 lbs and has over 1300 pages, and *PDR for Nutritional Supplements* weighs over 3 lbs and has more than 800 pages.

"I relied heavily on the PDRs during the research phase of writing my books. Without them, my projects would have greatly suffered."

- Bryan Rosner

We carry all three PDRs. Although PDR books are typically used by physicians, we feel that these resources are also essential for people interested in or recovering from chronic disease. For the supplements, herbs, and drugs included in the books, you will find the following information: Pharmacology, description and method of action, available trade names and brands, indications and usage, research summaries, dosage options, history of use, pharmacokinetics, and much more! Worth the money for years of faithful use.

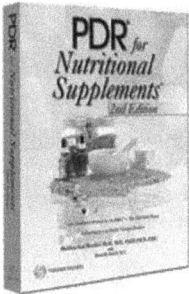

PDR for Nutritional Supplements   2nd Edition!

This PDR focuses on the following types of supplements:

- Vitamins
- Minerals
- Amino acids
- Hormones
- Lipids
- Glyconutrients
- Probiotics
- Proteins
- Many more!

"In a part of the health field not known for its devotion to rigorous science, [this book] brings to the practitioner and the curious patient a wealth of hard facts."

- Roger Guillemin, M.D., Ph.D., Nobel Laureate in Physiology and Medicine

Book • $69.50

The book also suggests supplements that can help reduce prescription drug side effects, has full-color photographs of various popular commercial formulations (and contact information for the associated suppliers), and so much more! Become educated instead of guessing which supplements to take.

Hardcover book, 11 x 9.3", 800 pages, $69.50

PDR for Herbal Medicines   4th Edition!

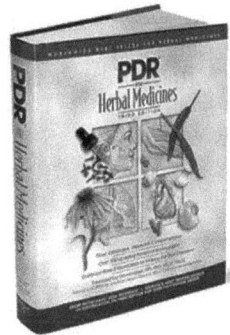

PDR for Herbal Medicines is very well organized and presents information on hundreds of common and uncommon herbs and herbal preparations. Indications and usage are examined with regard to homeopathy, Indian and Chinese medicine, and unproven (yet popular) applications.

In an area of healthcare so unstudied and vulnerable to hearsay and hype, this scientifically referenced book allows you to find out the real story behind the herbs lining the walls of your local health food store.

Use this reference before spending money on herbal products!

Book • $69.50

Hardcover book, 11 x 9.3", 1300 pages, $69.50

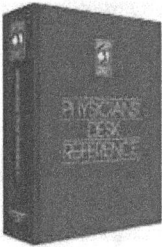

PDR for Prescription Drugs   Current Year's Edition!

With more than 3,000 pages, this is the most comprehensive and respected book in the world on over 4,000 drugs. Drugs are indexed by both brand and generic name (in the same convenient index) and also by manufacturer and product category. This PDR provides usage information and warnings, drug interactions, plus a detailed, full-color directory with descriptions and cross references for the drugs. A new format allows dramatically improved readability and easier access to the information you need now.

Book • $99.50

Hardcover book, 12.5 x 9.5", 3533 pages, $99.50

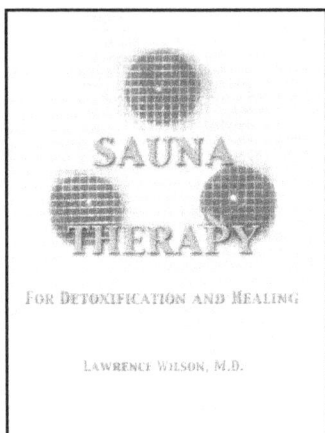

Sauna Therapy for Detoxification and Healing

By Lawrence Wilson, MD

This book provides a thorough yet articulate education on sauna therapy. It includes construction plans for a low-cost electric light sauna. The book is well referenced with an extensive bibliography.

Sauna therapy, especially with an electric light sauna, is one of the most powerful, safe and cost-effective methods of natural healing. It is especially important today due to extensive exposure to toxic metals and chemicals.

Fifteen chapters cover sauna benefits, physiological effects, protocols, cautions, healing reactions, and many other aspects of sauna therapy.

Book • $22.95

Dr. Wilson is an instructor of Biochemistry, Hair Mineral Analysis, Sauna Therapy and Jurisprudence at various colleges and universities including Yamuni Institute of the Healing Arts (Maurice, LA), University of Natural Medicine (Santa Fe, NM), Natural Healers Academy (Morristown, NJ), and Westbrook University (West Virginia). His books are used as textbooks at East-West School of Herbology and Ohio College of Natural Health. Go to www.LymeBook.com for free book excerpts!

Paperback book, 8.5 x 11", 167 pages, $22.95

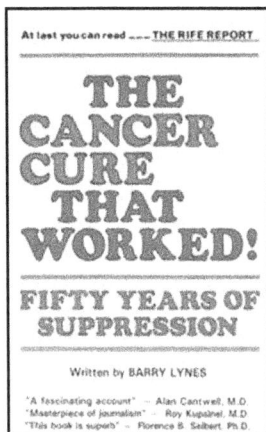

The Cancer Cure That Worked: Fifty Years of Suppression

At Last You Can Read... The Rife Report

By Barry Lynes

Investigative journalism at its best. Barry Lynes takes readers on an exciting journey into the life work of Royal Rife. We are now the official publisher of this book. Call or visit us online for wholesale terms.

Book • $19.95

Over 50,000 Copies Sold!

"A fascinating account..." **-Alan Cantwell, MD**

"This book is superb." **-Florence B. Seibert, PhD**

"Barry Lynes is one of the greatest health reporters in our country. With the assistance of John Crane, longtime friend and associate of Roy Rife, Barry has produced a masterpiece..." **-Roy Kupsinel, M.D., editor of *Health Consciousness Journal***

Paperback book, 5 x 8", 169 pages, $19.95

Rife Video Documentary
2-DVD Set, Produced by
Zero Zero Two Productions

Must-Have DVD set for your Rife technology education!

In 1999, a stack of forgotten audio tapes was discovered. On the tapes were the voices of several people at the center of the events which are the subject of this documentary: a revolutionary treatment for cancer and a practical cure for infectious disease.

The audio tapes were over 40 years old. The voices on them had almost faded, nearly losing key details of perhaps the most important medical story of the 20th Century.

But due to the efforts of the Kinnaman Foundation, the faded tapes have been restored and the voices on them recovered. So now, even though the participants have all passed away...

...they can finally tell their story.

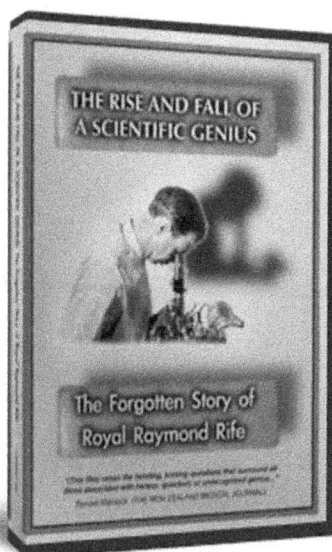

2-DVD Set • $39.95

"These videos are great. We show them at the Annual Rife International Health Conference."
-Richard Loyd, Ph.D.

"A mind-shifting experience for those of us indoctrinated with a conventional view of biology."
-Townsend Letter for Doctors and Patients

In the summer of 1934 at a special medical clinic in La Jolla, California, sixteen patients withering from terminal disease were given a new lease on life. It was the first controlled application of a new electronic treatment for cancer: the Beam Ray Machine.

Within ninety days all sixteen patients walked away from the clinic, signed-off by the attending doctors as cured.

What followed the incredible success of this revolutionary treatment was not a welcoming by the scientific community, but a sad tale of its ultimate suppression.

The Rise and Fall of a Scientific Genius documents the scientific ignorance, official corruption, and personal greed directed at the inventor of the Beam Ray Machine, Royal Raymond Rife, forcing him and his inventions out of the spotlight and into obscurity. **Just converted from VHS to DVD and completely updated.**

Includes bonus DVD with interviews and historical photographs! Produced in Canada.

Visit our website today to watch a FREE PREVIEW CLIP!

2 DVD-set, including bonus DVD, $39.95

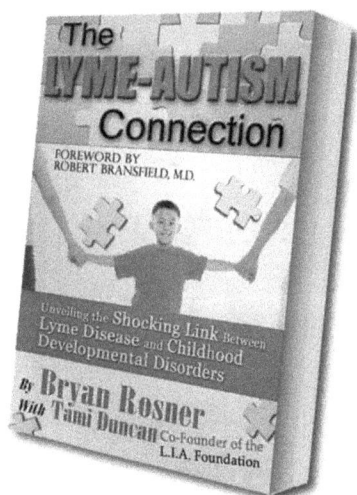

Book • $25.95

The Lyme-Autism Connection: Unveiling the Shocking Link Between Lyme Disease and Childhood Developmental Disorders

By Bryan Rosner & Tami Duncan

Did you know that Lyme disease may contribute to the onset of autism?

This book is an investigative report written by Bryan Rosner and Tami Duncan. Duncan is the co-founder of the *Lyme Induced Autism (LIA) Foundation*, and her son has an autism diagnosis.

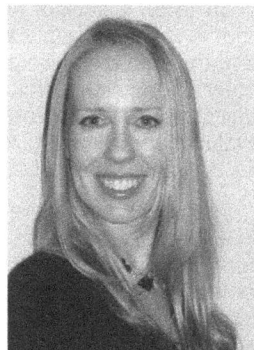

Tami Duncan, Co-Founder of the Lyme Induced Autism (LIA) Foundation

Awareness of the Lyme-autism connection is spreading rapidly, among both parents and practitioners. *Medical Hypothesis*, a scientific, peer-reviewed journal published by Elsevier, recently released an influential study entitled *The Association Between Tick-Borne Infections, Lyme Borreliosis and Autism Spectrum Disorders*. Here is an excerpt from the study:

> *"Chronic infectious diseases, including tick-borne infections such as Borrelia burgdorferi, may have direct effects, promote other infections, and create a weakened, sensitized and immunologically vulnerable state during fetal development and infancy, leading to increased vulnerability for developing autism spectrum disorders. An association between Lyme disease and other tick-borne infections and autistic symptoms has been noted by numerous clinicians and parents."*

—Medical Hypothesis Journal.
Article Authors: Robert C. Bransfield, M.D., Jeffrey S. Wulfman, M.D., William T. Harvey, M.D., Anju I. Usman, M.D.

Nationwide, 1 out of 150 children are diagnosed with Autism Spectrum Disorder (ASD), and the LIA Foundation has discovered that many of these children test positive for Lyme disease/Borrelia related complex—yet most children in this scenario never receive appropriate medical attention. This book answers many difficult questions: How can infants contract Lyme disease if autism begins before birth, precluding the opportunity for a tick bite? Is there a statistical correlation between the incidences of Lyme disease and autism worldwide? Do autistic children respond to Lyme disease treatment? What does the medical community say about this connection? Do the mothers of affected children exhibit symptoms? **Find out in this book.**

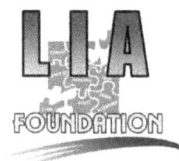

Paperback book, 6x9", 287 pages, $25.95

Dietrich Klinghardt, M.D., Ph.D.
"Fundamental Teachings"
5-DVD Set

Includes Disc Exclusively For Lyme Disease!

Dietrich Klinghardt, M.D., Ph.D. is a legendary healer known for discovering and refining many of the cutting-edge treatment protocols used for a variety of chronic health problems including Lyme disease, autism and mercury poisoning.

Now you can find out all about this doctor's treatment methods from the privacy of your own home! This 5-DVD set includes the following DVDs:

- **DISC 1**: The Five Levels of Healing and the Seven Factors

- **DISC 2**: Autonomic Response Testing and Demonstration

- **DISC 3**: Heavy Metal Toxicity and Neurotoxin Elimination / Electrosmog

- **DISC 4**: Lyme disease and Chronic Illness

- **DISC 5**: Psycho-Emotional Issues in Chronic Illness & Addressing Underlying Causes

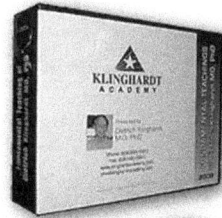

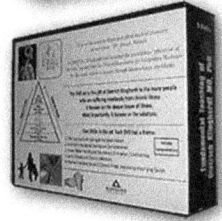

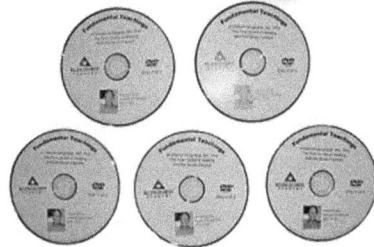

5-DVD Set • $125

Dr. Dietrich Klinghardt is one of the most important contributors to modern integrative treatment for Lyme disease and related medical conditions. This comprehensive DVD set is a must-have addition to your educational library.

5-DVD Set, $125

Our catalog has space limitations, but our website does not! Visit www.LymeBook.com to see even more exciting products.

Don't Miss These New Books & DVDs, Available Online:
- Babesia Update by James Schaller, M.D.
- Bryan Rosner's Anti-Lyme Journal/Newsletter
- Cure Unknown, by Pamela Weintraub
- The Experts of Lyme Disease, by Sue Vogan
- The Lyme Disease Solution, by Ken Singleton, M.D.
- **Lots of Free Chapters and Excerpts Online!**

Don't use the internet? No problem, just call (530) 573-0190.

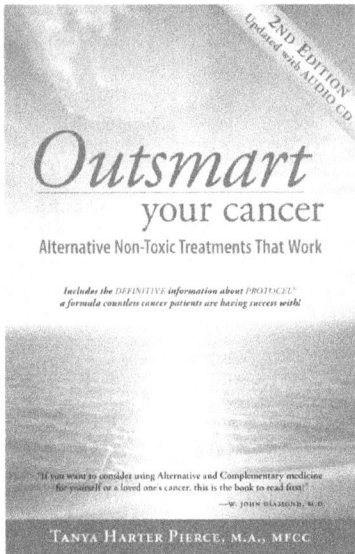

2nd Edition! **Outsmart Your Cancer: Alternative Non-Toxic Treatments That Work   By Tanya Harter Pierce**

Why BLUDGEON cancer to death with common conventional treatments that can be toxic and harmful to your entire body?

When you OUTSMART your cancer, only the cancer cells die — NOT your healthy cells! *OUTSMART YOUR CANCER: Alternative Non-Toxic Treatments That Work* is an easy guide to successful non-toxic treatments for cancer that you can obtain right now! In it, you will read real-life stories of people who have completely recovered from their advanced or late-stage lung cancer, breast cancer, prostate cancer, kidney cancer, brain cancer, childhood leukemia, and other types of cancer using effective non-toxic approaches.

Book and Audio CD • $26.95

Plus, *OUTSMART YOUR CANCER* is one of the few books in print today that gives a complete description of the amazing formula called "Protocel," which has produced incredible cancer recoveries over the past 20 years. **A supporting audio CD is included with this book**.

Paperback book, 6 x 9", 437 pages, with audio CD, $26.95

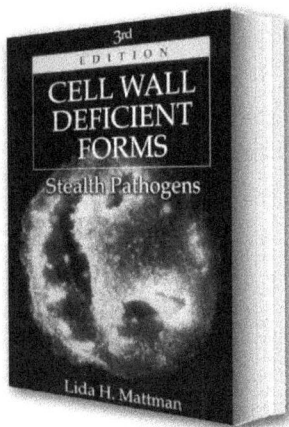

Cell Wall Deficient Forms: Stealth Pathogens

By Lida Mattman, Ph.D.

This is one of the most influential infectious disease textbook of the century. Dr. Mattman, who earned a Ph.D. in immunology from Yale University, describes her discovery that a certain type of pathogen lacking a cell wall is the root cause of many of today's "incurable" and mysterious chronic diseases. Dr. Mattman's research is the foundation of our current understanding of Lyme disease, and her work led to many of the Lyme protocols used today (such as the Marshall Protocol, as well as modern LLMD antibiotic treatment strategy). Color illustrations and meticulously referenced breakthrough principles cover the pages of this book. A must have for all serious students of chronic, elusive infectious disease.

Hardcover Book • $169.95

Hardcover book, 7.5 x 10.5", 416 pages, $169.95

Order by Phone: (866) 476-7637

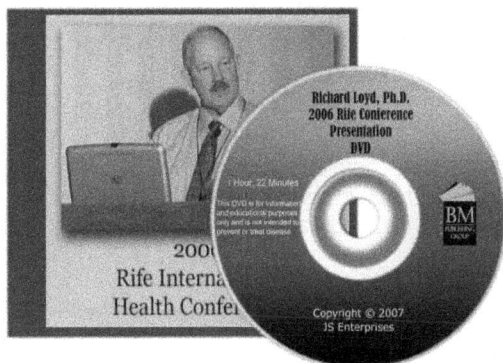

DVD • $24.50

Richard Loyd, Ph.D., presents at the Rife International Health Conference in Seattle

Watch this DVD to gain a better understanding of the technical details of rife technology.

Dr. Loyd, who earned a Ph.D. in nutrition, has researched and experimented with numerous electrotherapeutic devices, including the Rife/Bare unit, various EMEM machines, F-Scan, BioRay, magnetic pulsers, Doug Machine, and more. Dr. Loyd also has a wealth of knowledge in the use of herbs and supplements to support Rife electromagnetics.

By watching this DVD, you will discover the nuts and bolts of some very important, yet little known, principles of rife machine operation, including:

- Gating, sweeping, session time
- Square vs. sine wave
- DC vs. AC frequencies
- Duty cycle
- Octaves and scalar octaves
- Voltage variations and radio frequencies
- Explanation of the spark gap
- Contact vs. radiant mode
- Stainless vs. copper contacts
- A unique look at various frequency devices

DVD, 57 minutes, $24.50

Under Our Skin:
Lyme Disease Documentary Film

A gripping tale of microbes, medicine & money, UNDER OUR SKIN exposes the hidden story of Lyme disease, one of the most serious and controversial epidemics of our time. Each year, thousands go undiagnosed or misdiagnosed, often told that their symptoms are all in their head. Following the stories of patients and physicians fighting for their lives and livelihoods, the film brings into focus a haunting picture of the health care system and a medical establishment all too willing to put profits ahead of patients.

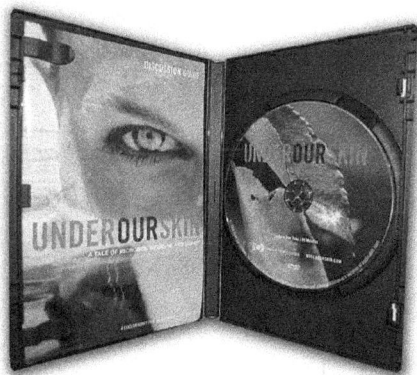

DVD • $34.95

Bonus Features: 32-page discussion guidebook, one hour of bonus footage, director's commentary, and much more! **FOR HOME USE ONLY**

DVD with bonus features, 104 minutes, $34.95 *MUST SEE!*

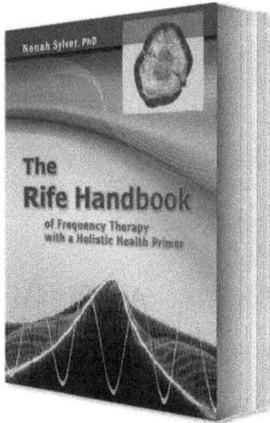

www.ingramcontent.com/pod-product-compliance
Lightning Source LLC
Chambersburg PA
CBHW080132270326
41926CB00021B/4447